Current Clinical Practice

Series Editor

Tommy Koonce
Family Medicine
University of North Carolina at Chapel Hill
Chapel Hill, USA

More information about this series at http://www.springer.com/series/7633

Paul Lyons • Nathan McLaughlin

Obstetrics in Family Medicine

A Practical Guide

Third Edition

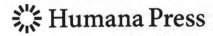
Humana Press

Paul Lyons
School of Medicine
California University of Science
and Medicine
San Bernardino, CA
USA

Nathan McLaughlin
School of Medicine
University of California
Riverside, CA
USA

Current Clinical Practice
ISBN 978-3-030-39887-3   ISBN 978-3-030-39888-0   (eBook)
https://doi.org/10.1007/978-3-030-39888-0

This Humana imprint is published by the registered company Springer Nature Switzerland AG
The registered company address is: Gewerbestrasse 11, 6330 Cham, Switzerland

Preface

One of the joys of working in obstetrics is the privilege of being present as the current generation gives rise to the next generation. It is, of course, not the transition in its entirety, but it is a seminal moment in the journey. Over the years, I have been blessed to be present with thousands of women and their families at precisely that moment, to share in that journey and all its associated emotions—hope, fear, anxiety, disappointment (on occasion), and joy.

When I wrote the first edition of this textbook, I was in the midst of that journey in my own life with a young career and an even younger family. With this third edition, my children are now grown, my professional life has evolved, and I am pleased to both recognize and acknowledge those changes. I am grateful to my wife, Cynthia, who continues to provide support and inspiration, and to my two children, Devin and Dylan, now delightful young adults, who give me great hope for and faith in the next generation.

With this edition I am pleased to share in generational change, in the professional sense as well. As my professional life has less direct involvement in delivery of obstetrical patient care, I have become in some ways the audience for as much as the author of this text, "all of us who care for women may find it useful to have a reference that addresses key clinical issues in this important element of women's health," as I noted in the preface to the second edition. In that transition, I have been blessed to be present with young professionals who represent the future such care. I am pleased to share the creation of this edition with Dr. Nathan McLaughlin, a delightful young physician who gives me great hope for and faith in what comes next.

San Bernardino, CA, USA   Paul Lyons

Preface

Having great mentorship is instrumental to success and can greatly affect one's trajectory in life. I am lucky to have had a sizeable number of influential mentors that have shaped my education and career. In medical school, it was Dr. Michelle Whitehurst-Cook and Dr. Steve Crossman providing shining examples of what family physicians could be. During residency training Dr. Evelyn Figueroa and Dr. Mark Potter were there to guide me into full-spectrum family medicine including obstetrics, which has enriched my life greatly. I am indebted to those listed above and countless others who have helped to bring me to where I am today.

Over the past 6 years, Dr. Paul Lyons has provided me with mentorship, support, guidance, and opportunity that I could only dream of. The most recent opportunity was in the form of this book. Being asked to help write this third edition of *Obstetrics in Family Medicine: A Practical Guide* is a great honor, and honestly one that I never expected. Dr. Lyons' casual belief in me bolstered my confidence to take on a task that was beyond anything I had done before. Despite his constant assertions that he really doesn't do anything, his impact on me has been immense. I can only hope to provide others with the guidance and support that my mentors have given to me, for without that support I truly would not be where I am today.

Most importantly, I would like to thank my loving wife, Whitney Sullivan-Lewis, MD, for providing me with endless support and reassurance that allow me to have a fulfilling life and career. She is an amazing doctor, wife, and mother, and I should tell her this more often than I do. Lastly, all of my love and affection to my two daughters, Virginia and Josephine, who love me, despite my imperfections, and serve as a constant reminder of what is truly important in life.

Riverside, CA, USA   Nathan McLaughlin

Contents

Part I   Preconception and Prenatal Care

1   Physiology 3
    Background.. 3
    Physiology of Menstruation 4
    Physiology of Fertility 5
        Hypothalamic Function....................................... 5
        Pituitary Function 6
        Ovulation... 6
    Physiology of Pregnancy 7
        Cardiovascular Changes 8
        Renal/Urinary Changes....................................... 8
        Gastrointestinal Changes 9
        Hematological Changes 9

2   Preconception Counseling 11
    Background.. 11
        The Patient 12
        The Environment... 13
    Getting Started 13
    Screening.. 14
    Education 15
    Intervention... 16

3   Prenatal Care.. 19
    Background.. 20
    Key Domains of Prenatal Information 21
    Frequency of Prenatal Visits 22
        The First Prenatal Visit 22
        History... 22
    Physical Examination 25
    Laboratory and Diagnostic Testing................................ 25

Estimating Gestational Age.   26
Laboratory Testing   27
Treatment and Follow-Up.   27
    Follow-Up Prenatal Visits.   27
Interval History and Physical Exam   28
    Structure of Prenatal Visits   28
Interval Laboratory and Diagnostic Studies   29

4   Medications in Pregnancy   31
    Background.   32
    General Principles of Medication Use in Pregnancy   32
        Chronic Medical Conditions.   32
        Acute Medical Conditions   33
        Acute Obstetrical Conditions   34
        Therapeutic Categories and Considerations   34
    Proven Human Teratogens   35
    Special Considerations   36
        Tobacco.   36
        Alcohol.   37
        Illicit Drugs.   37
    Over-the-Counter Medications   37
        OTC Pain Medications   38
    Acetaminophen.   38
    Aspirin.   38
    Nonsteroidal Anti-inflammatory Drugs   39
        OTC Cough/Cold/Allergy Medications   39
    Antihistamines   39
    Decongestants.   39
    Cough Medications.   40

5   Vaccines in Pregnancy   41
    Background.   41
    Infectious Diseases in Pregnancy   42
    Vaccines Recommended in All Pregnancies.   42
        Influenza   42
        Tetanus, Diphtheria, and Pertussis (Tdap)   43
    Vaccines to Be Considered Based on Risk vs. Benefit.   43
        Hepatitis A   43
        Yellow Fever.   43
        Meningococcal (B)   43
    Vaccines for Use if Indicated   44
    Vaccines Contraindicated in Pregnancy   44

Part II   Complications in Pregnancy

**6   Dysmorphic Growth and Genetic
   Abnormalities**   47
   Background   47
   History   48
   Physical Examination   49
   Diagnosis   49
   Obstetrical Screening Tests   50
      What Is Measured   50
      What Is Detected   50
      Confirmation/Follow-Up   51
      Amniocentesis   51
      Chorionic Villus Sampling   52

7   Intrauterine Growth Restriction   53
   Background   53
   Risk Factors   55
      Fetal–Genetic Factors   55
      Uterine–Environmental Factors   55
      Maternal Factors   56
      Toxic Exposures   56
      Constitutional Factors   57
   Complications of Growth Restriction   57
   Antenatal Tracking and Diagnosis   57
   Screening for Risks   59
   Diagnosis   60
   Management   60
      Risk Reduction   60

8   Preterm Labor   63
   Background   64
   Factors Associated with Preterm Labor   64
   Preconception Factor   65
      Environmental Factors   65
      Patient-Related Factors   65
   Postconception Factors   65
   Diagnosis   66
   Intake Assessment   66
      History   66
      Physical Examination   67
      Laboratory Studies   67

Management   67
Management Prior to 34 Weeks' Gestation   69
Management at 34–37 Weeks   70
Assessment of Fetal Lung Maturity   70
Lecithin-to-Sphingomyelin Ratio   71
Phosphatidylglycerol   71
Additional Tests   71

9 Premature Rupture of Membranes   73
Background   73
Diagnosis   74
History   74
Physical Examination   75
Laboratory   76
Management   77
Management at Term   78
Preterm Management   78

10 Early Pregnancy Bleeding   79
Background   80
General Approach to Early Pregnancy Bleeding Per Vagina   80
History   81
Physical Examination   81
Ultrasound   83
Laboratory Studies   83
Ectopic Pregnancy   84
Background   84
Diagnosis   84
Management   85
Spontaneous Abortion   86
Background   86
Diagnosis   87
Management   88

11 Late-Pregnancy Bleeding   91
Background   92
General Approach to Late-Pregnancy Bleeding Per Vagina   92
History   94
Ultrasound   94
Physical Examination   95
Laboratory Studies   95
Placenta Previa   95
Background   95
History   96
Ultrasound Examination   96
Physical Examination   96

Laboratory Studies 96
Management 97
Management at Term 97
Preterm Management 97
Abruptio Placenta 97
Background 97
History 98
Ultrasound 98
Physical Examination 98
Laboratory Studies 99
Management 99

12 **Recurrent Pregnancy Loss** 101
Background 101
Diagnosis 103
Management 103
History 103
Physical Examination 104
Diagnostic Studies 104

13 **Rh Isoimmunization** 107
Background 107
Fetal Consequences of Isoimmunization 108
Newborn Consequences of Isoimmunization 109
Diagnosis 109
History 109
Physical Examination 109
Diagnostic Studies 109
Management Prior to Isoimmunization 110
Management of Pregnancies with Rh-Sensitized Mothers 110
Amniotic Fluid Assessment 112
Ultrasonography 112
Percutaneous Umbilical Blood Sampling 112

14 **Infection in Pregnancy** 113
Background 114
Symptoms of Infection in Pregnancy 115
Maternal Infection 115
Fetal Infection 116
Antibiotic Use in Pregnancy 117
Sulfonamides 117
Fluoroquinolones 118
Aminoglycosides 118
Vaginitis/Vaginosis 118
Background 118
History 119

Physical Examination 119
Laboratory Studies 119
pH *Testing* 120
KOH *Whiff* 120
Microscopic Examination 120
Treatment 120
Bacterial Vaginosis 120
Trichomoniasis 121
Yeast Vaginitis 121
Gonorrhea/Chlamydia 121
Urinary Tract Infections 122
Background 122
Diagnosis 122
History 122
Physical Examination 123
Laboratory Examination 123
Treatment 123
Group B Strep 124
Background 124
Diagnosis 124
Universal Screening 125
Treatment 125

15   Hypertension in Pregnancy 127
Background 128
Diagnosis 128
Diagnostic Criteria 128
History 130
Physical Examination 130
Laboratory Studies 130
Management 131
Chronic Hypertension 131
Pre-eclampsia 131
Prevention 131
Management 131
Seizure Prevention 133
Postpartum Management 134

16   Diabetes in Pregnancy 135
Background 135
Diagnosis 136
Pregestational Diabetes 137
Management 137
Management in Pregnancy 138
Diet 138
Insulin 139

Oral Hypoglycemics... 139
Blood Sugar Monitoring...................................... 139
Gestational Diabetes... 140
    Preconception Management 140
Management in Pregnancy 140
Management in Labor.. 141
Postpartum Management 141

17 HIV in Pregnancy.. 143
Preconception Counseling 144
Initial Pregnancy Evaluation................................. 144
Antiretroviral Use in Pregnancy 145
Intrapartum Management 146
Postpartum Management 147

18 Multigestational Pregnancy............................ 149
Background.. 149
Diagnosis... 151
    History.. 152
    Physical Examination 152
    Laboratory and Diagnostic Studies..................... 152
    Management 152
        Prenatal Care... 152
        Labor and Delivery 153

19 Postdates Pregnancy.................................... 155
Background.. 155
Diagnosis... 156
    History.. 156
    Physical Examination 157
    Diagnostic Studies 157
    Management 157
    Assessment of Fetal Well-Being......................... 157
Fetal Kick Count... 158
Amniotic Fluid Volume.. 159
Ultrasound Estimate of Fetal Weight 159
Nonstress Test.. 159
Contraction Stress Test 159
Biophysical Profile 160

Part III   Labor and Delivery

20 Normal Labor 163
Background.. 163
Prelabor.. 164
Labor... 164
Assessment 165

      History... 165
      Physical Examination 165
   Dilation.. 166
   Effacement 166
   Station... 166
   Presentation.. 166
   Laboratory Studies 167
   Management 167

21 Induction and Augmentation 169
   Background.. 169
   Preparation 169
      Pharmacological Options 170
      Mechanical Options 171
   Induction... 171

22 Pain Management in Labor 173
   Background.. 173
   Nonpharmacological Management................................ 174
   Pharmacological Management 174
      Narcotic Analgesia 174
      Local Anesthesia.. 175
      Epidural–Spinal Anesthesia 175

Part IV Complications of Labor and Delivery

23 Assisted Delivery.. 179
   Background.. 179
   Forceps Delivery.. 180
      Use of Forceps 181
   Vacuum-Assisted Delivery 181
   Cesarean Section.. 182

24 Prolonged Labor 183
   Background.. 183
   Complications of Labor 184
      Prolonged Latent-Phase Labor 184
   History... 185
   Physical Examination 185
   Laboratory/Diagnostic Studies 185
   Management 185
      Failure to Dilate/Efface.................................. 186
   History... 186
   Physical Examination 186
   Laboratory/Diagnostic Studies 187
   Management 187
      Failure to Descend 188

25 Shoulder Dystocia 189
     Background 189
     Diagnosis 190
     Management 191

26 Malpresentation 193
     Background 193
     Occiput Positions 194
         Diagnosis 194
         Management 194
     Nonoccipital Presentations 194
     Breech Presentation 195
     Compound Presentation 196

27 Fetal Heart Rate Monitoring 197
     Background 197
         Normal Fetal Heart Tracings 198
     Evaluation of Fetal Heart Rate Baseline 198
         Tachycardia 199
         Bradycardia 199
     Evaluation of Fetal Heart Rate Variability 199
         Acceleration 199
         Early Deceleration 200
         Variable Deceleration 200
         Late Decelerations 200
     Classification of Electronic Fetal Monitoring 201

28 Maternal Fever in Labor 203
     Background 203
     Diagnosis 204
         History 204
         Physical Examination 204
         Diagnostic Studies 205
     Management 205

29 Postpartum Hemorrhage 207
     Background 208
     Complications Causing Hemorrhage 208
         Uterine Atony 208
         Lacerations 209
         Retained Placenta 209
         Coagulopathy 209
         Uterine Inversion 209
     Diagnosis 209
     Management 210
         Laceration 210
         Persistent Bleeding 211

30   Perineal Laceration and Episiotomy 213
       Episiotomy 213
          Background 213
       Procedure 214
       Perineal Laceration 214
          Background 214
       Diagnosis 214
          History 214
       Physical Examination 215
       Management 215

Part V   Postpartum Management

31   Newborn Evaluation 219
       Background 220
       The Examination 220
          History 220
          Physical Examination 220
       Vital Signs 220
       General Observation 221
       Head and Neck 221
       Eyes 221
       Cardiovascular 221
       Pulmonary/Thoracic 222
       Abdomen 222
       Genital Examination 222
       Anus 222
       Spine 222
       Skin 223
       Extremities 223
       Neurologic 223
          Laboratory and Diagnostic Studies 223
          Vaccination 224

32   Routine Hospital Postpartum Management 225
       Background 225
       Postpartum Day 1 226
          History 226
          Physical Examination 226
          Laboratory Studies 227
       Management 227
       Postpartum Day 2 228
          History 228
          Physical Examination 228

          Laboratory Studies   229
          Management   229

33   Complications of the Hospital Postpartum Period   231
          Background.   231
          Persistent Postpartum Hemorrhage.   231
          Hypertension.   232
          Thromboembolic Disease   232
          Fever   232
          Infection   233
               Endometritis   233
               Urinary Tract Infections   234

34   Postpartum Clinic Visit.   235
          Background.   235
          Postpartum Depression   236
          Infant Care and Feeding   236
          Sexuality/Relationships.   237
          Vaginal Bleeding.   237
          Self-Care   237
          Management of Complications.   238
               Hypertensive Disorders.   238
               Gestational Diabetes   238

Index.   239

Part I
Preconception and Prenatal Care

Chapter 1
Physiology

Contents

Background... 3
Physiology of Menstruation.. 4
Physiology of Fertility.. 5
    Hypothalamic Function... 5
    Pituitary Function... 6
    Ovulation... 6
Physiology of Pregnancy.. 7
    Cardiovascular Changes.. 8
    Renal/Urinary Changes... 8
    Gastrointestinal Changes... 9
    Hematological Changes... 9

> **Key Points**
> 1. The menstrual cycle can be considered a comprehensive physiological adaptation for potential pregnancy.
> 2. Normal menstrual cycles last 21–45 days (average 28 days), counted from the first day of menstrual bleeding.
> 3. Physiological adaptations of pregnancy affect most major organ systems including cardiac, renal, gastrointestinal, and endocrine systems.

Background

Although most patients will not present to their providers with questions concerning the specifics of reproductive physiology, the care and management of pregnant patients begin with an understanding of the physiological environment in which pregnancy occurs (or in some instances, does not occur). Many women's health providers will face questions concerning menstrual function prior to caring for a patient's obstetrical needs. Conversely, routine gynecological care may provide an opportunity to begin discussions of pregnancy planning and preconception counseling. For many women, a "routine" gynecological examination is the primary point of contact with the health-care system early in life. For this reason, all providers who care for women should have some understanding of normal reproductive physiological function. A brief overview of menstruation, fertility, and pregnancy follows.

Physiology of Menstruation

Menstruation represents the cyclical physiological preparation for potential pregnancy, followed by removal of endometrial contents if pregnancy does not occur. Most women of reproductive age are familiar with menstruation. The average age of menarche in the United States is approximately 11.5 years. Most menstrual cycles are anovulatory in the first year following menarche and may remain irregularly ovulatory for up to 3 years (although women and providers should be aware that ovulation and/or pregnancy may occur). For the next three to four decades, most women will menstruate every 21–35 days (average 28 ± 7 days). Bleeding is variable but generally lasts 3–5 days (1–7 days may be considered normal) and is of variable intensity (but generally less than 3 oz or 90 cm^3).

Although generally considered an ovarian and uterine phenomenon, the normal menstrual cycle may be considered as a comprehensive physiological adaptation in preparation for possible pregnancy. In addition to the uterine and ovarian changes described here, changes can be noted in the cervix, vagina, breast, and core body temperature. The cervical mucus becomes thinner with increased pH to facilitate entry of sperm. Vaginal epithelial cells also undergo change. Mammary ducts proliferate under estrogen and progesterone stimulation, which may lead to breast swelling and tenderness. A small spike in basal body temperature can be seen at the time of ovulation. This observation has contributed to the use of basal body monitoring in fertility management.

Physiologically, bleeding represents the end of one cycle. From the perspective of the patient and the provider, however, bleeding is the most easily identified aspect of the menstrual cycle and is, therefore, used to mark the beginning of each cycle. The first day of menstrual bleeding is day 1 with each day numbered sequentially through the last day prior to the recurrence of bleeding. Each menstrual cycle can be divided into two-halves that differ in hormonal and physiological events. In a typical or average menstrual cycle, each half is approximately 14 days in duration.

The first half of each menstrual cycle is marked by endometrial proliferation and follicular development. In the first week of each menstrual cycle, multiple follicles enlarge. At approximately 1 week, a single follicle becomes dominant and the others involute, becoming atretic. The dominant follicle will, with appropriate hormonal regulation, continue to develop and will eventually rupture releasing an ovum for possible fertilization. With release of the ovum on day 14, the follicle undergoes a series of stereotypic changes filling with blood, granulose, and thecal cell proliferation and displacement of blood by luteal cells (corpus luteum). The luteal cells produce progesterone, which serves to stabilize the thickened endometrium through the second half of the menstrual cycle. The period of follicle development is referred to as the follicular phase. The period of luteal production of progesterone is referred to as the luteal phase.

Follicular development in the first half of each menstrual cycle is marked by follicular production of estrogen and endometrial proliferation in anticipation of possible implantation of a fertilized ovum. This generally occurs late in the first week and throughout the second week of the menstrual cycle. The first half of the menstrual cycle is, for this reason, sometimes referred to as the proliferative phase. With ovulation and luteal production of estrogen and progesterone, uterine glands become active, secreting clear fluid. This phase is referred to as the secretory phase. The endometrium will remain stable and secretory for as long as the progesterone stimulation continues.

If fertilization fails to occur, the corpus luteum will lose function beginning in the second half of the fourth week (corpus albicans). With the loss of hormonal support, endometrial thinning and localized necrosis lead to sloughing of the proliferative portion of the endometrial lining and the onset of menses. Until menopause, this cycle will repeat more or less regularly each month.

Physiology of Fertility

The hormonal changes just described relate to preparation for release of the ovum and subsequent fertilization by sperm. As noted, however, these menstrual changes may occur in the absence of ovulation. In addition, under normal physiological conditions, pregnancy requires the presence of functional sperm in sufficient quantity to ensure fertilization of the released ovum.

In women, the release of an ovum is under the control of the hypothalamic–pituitary–ovarian endocrinological axis. Each of these components must function normally to ensure ovum release. Two pituitary hormones, in particular, are critical to normal ovulatory cycles—follicle-stimulating hormone (FSH) and luteinizing hormone (LH).

Hypothalamic Function

Release of pituitary hormones depends on hypothalamic stimulation. The hypothalamus is responsible for stimulation of a variety of pituitary hormones, and hypothalamic dysfunction may manifest with altered fertility or a variety of other endocrinological signs or symptoms. In addition to pituitary stimulation, the hypothalamus is responsible for direct release of oxytocin (of import at the time of labor).

In relation to fertility, hypothalamic release of gonadotropin-releasing hormone (GnRH) stimulates the anterior pituitary production of FSH and LH. GnRH is produced in the hypothalamus and released directly to the pituitary via local blood vessels. Release of GnRH is episodic in brief, timed bursts. Although GnRH cannot be measured directly, pulsatile GnRH release results in pulsatile release of LH which can be measured providing indirect evidence of hypothalamic function. Failure to maintain this episodic release will inhibit pituitary stimulation, probably secondary to downregulation of pituitary receptors. Disruption of the timing of the episodic release will also impair fertility by disrupting the appropriate timing of FSH and LH stimulation of the ovary. In addition, appropriately episodic and timed GnRH stimulates pituitary GnRh receptors enhancing sensitivity at mid-cycle and facilitating a surge in LH at the time of ovulation.

Pituitary Function

As with the hypothalamus, the pituitary is responsible for the release of several hormones regulating a variety of physiological functions. In relation to fertility, the two key hormones are the gonadotropins, FSH and LH. These two agents are released cyclically and in a pulsatile fashion in response to GnRH stimulation. Together they are responsible for regulation of ovarian hormonal secretion. Pituitary release of FSH and LH is also regulated by ovarian hormone release. Ovarian release of estradiol results in negative feedback (inhibition) of FSH release and positive feedback (stimulation) of LH release.

FSH, as the name implies, is responsible for stimulating early follicle development within the ovary. LH fosters ovarian production of estrogen and progesterone from the corpus luteum. In conjunction with LH, FSH is also responsible for terminal maturation. At the point of maturation, a surge in LH levels precipitates follicular rupture and ovum release.

Ovulation

Early in the menstrual cycle, FSH levels are slightly elevated (stimulating follicular development), and LH levels are low. In this phase of the menstrual cycle, estrogen serves an inhibitory role on LH. GnRH stimulation of the pituitary continues, and the sensitivity of the pituitary is enhanced. Approximately 2 days prior to ovulation, the estrogen inhibition is reversed, becoming stimulatory, and a positive feedback loop is established. Approximately 8–10 h prior to ovulation, LH levels reach a peak

(LH surge). Ovulation then occurs. Following ovulation, estrogen once again becomes inhibitory and, in conjunction with elevated progesterone levels, serves to inhibit LH and FSH levels in the second half of the menstrual cycle.

Physiology of Pregnancy

The physiological changes associated with pregnancy are numerous, and the full scope of such changes is beyond the scope of this text. Common physiological changes with pregnancy are summarized in Table 1.1. Recognition of normal physiological changes

Table 1.1 Physiological changes of pregnancy	Cardiovascular
	Cardiac enlargement
	Increased cardiac output
	Systolic flow murmur
	Decreased venous return
	Decreased peripheral vascular resistance
	Decreased blood pressure
	Increased blood flow to the uterus, kidneys, skin, breasts
	Renal/urinary
	Increased urinary stasis
	Increased urinary system volume
	Kidney enlargement
	Renal pelvis dilatation
	Ureteral elongation
	Increased bladder capacity
	Increased glomerular filtration rate
	Elevation of renin, aldosterone, angiotensin
	Glucosuria
	Gastrointestinal
	Early satiety
	Nausea, vomiting
	Constipation
	Gingival hypertrophy
	Progression of periodontal disease
	Decreased gastric emptying
	Relaxation of lower esophageal sphincter
	Hematological
	Increased red blood cell volume
	Anemia
	Leukocytosis

is necessary not only to understand normal function while pregnant but also to facilitate recognition of physiological abnormalities that lie outside the normal range.

Cardiovascular Changes

Pregnancy can be considered an adaptive high-volume, hyperdynamic cardiovascular state. Increased volume, a newly developed peripheral vascular bed, and anatomic changes associated with an enlarging uterus all serve to alter normal cardiovascular status. The heart, itself, enlarges, and cardiac output increases by nearly 50%. This increased output is initially facilitated by an increase in cardiac volume and subsequently by an increase in heart rate. The increase in output reaches a peak near the end of the second trimester and then remains stable until the end of pregnancy.

The increase in volume may lead to increased flow turbulence within the heart. This turbulence may be apparent clinically as a systolic ejection murmur. Such a murmur will manifest in 80–90% of all pregnant women. This murmur is a normal physiological finding and does not warrant further cardiovascular investigation.

Vascular changes are also common in pregnancy. With an increase in uterine size, venous return via the inferior vena cava may be directly impaired. Placing the patient in the left lateral recumbent position may alleviate the direct pressure of the uterus on the vena cava and facilitate enhanced venous return. The direct compression of venous return from the lower extremities may lead to peripheral edema. Peripheral vascular resistance declines with pregnancy as maternal cardiac output increases. Compensatory venous response to rapid position changes may also be impaired in pregnancy causing light-headedness or dizziness with rapid positional changes. Blood pressure often declines slightly (approximately 10 mmHg diastolic) with a nadir in the second trimester and a slight rise (to near prepregnant levels) near the end of pregnancy.

Blood flow is altered in pregnancy as well. The most obvious change is the increase in uterine blood flow with the development of the uteroplacental vascular bed. Blood flow through this vascular bed is facilitated by vascular resistance that is low relative to the overall peripheral vascular resistance. In addition to increased blood flow to the uterus, maternal blood flow is increased to the kidneys, breast, and extremities (including increased flow to the skin). Although concern has been raised that exercise may divert blood flow from these key areas to muscles, this has generally not been found to be clinically significant except for women who significantly increase their activity level from their prepregnancy baseline. A reasonable recommendation would be that women may continue exercise through pregnancy at a level not to exceed their usual degree of exertion.

Renal/Urinary Changes

Pregnancy is marked by an increase in urinary stasis. The direct impingement of the uterus and fetus on the bladder contributes to this effect as do anatomic changes within the urinary tract. Kidneys enlarge, the renal pelvis dilates, and the course of the ureter elongates contributing to increased volume within the urinary tract. This increased volume in turn contributes to an increase in post-void residual urine within the tract and subsequent stasis.

Renal function is also changed in pregnancy. A combination of hormonal modulation with increased plasma volume leads to an increase of nearly 50% in the glomerular filtration rate. Renin, angiotensin, and aldosterone levels are all elevated in pregnancy. Despite this increase in glomerular filtration, urinary output is not increased during pregnancy. Although many patients will report increased urinary frequency, the total output volume remains similar to the prepregnancy levels (the functional capacity of the bladder is, in fact, increased in pregnancy with a total capacity of approximately 1.5 L). Aldosterone-mediated sodium resorption in turn leads to fluid resorption and maintenance of intravascular homeostasis. Increased renal filtration does lead to increased creatinine clearance and a concomitant reduction in serum creatinine levels (along with decreased blood urea nitrogen levels). Sporadic glucosuria is a common finding in pregnancy and may be an artifact of increased glomerular filtration.

Gastrointestinal Changes

Gastrointestinal (GI) symptoms are among the most common complaints of pregnancy. Early in pregnancy nausea and vomiting are often reported. Later in pregnancy, early satiety and constipation are both commonly observed. Although these symptoms are generally not related to specific changes within the GI tract, some physiological alterations are noted with pregnancy. Gingival hypertrophy and worsening of gingival disease have both been reported. Some investigators have suggested a possible link between periodontal disease and an increased risk of preterm labor, although the results are preliminary and inconclusive. GI motility is decreased, including a decrease in gastric emptying and increased transit time through the large intestine. Decreased gastric emptying combined with relaxation of the terminal portion of the esophagus may lead to an increase in reports of gastroesophageal reflux symptoms. This may be exacerbated late in pregnancy as the uterus increasingly displaces the stomach upward.

Hematological Changes

Pregnancy is associated with a variety of changes in hematological status. With an increase in intravascular volume, patients also experience an increase in red cell volume. This increase in red cell volume, in turn, increases the patient's need for iron. With inadequate dietary iron (either from food or supplementation), many pregnant patients will develop an iron deficiency anemia with the usual change in red cell indices (decreased mean corpuscular volume and decreased mean corpuscular hemoglobin content). An increase in blood leukocytes is common in pregnancy. Levels rise throughout pregnancy and peak during labor. Such a rise in white blood cells may make determination of infection more complicated.

Chapter 2
Preconception Counseling

Contents

Background... 11
   The Patient... 12
   The Environment... 13
Getting Started.. 13
Screening... 14
Education... 15
Intervention... 16

Key Points

1. Preconception counseling is a medical evaluation and intervention performed prior to conception with the expectation that the course and outcome of subsequent pregnancies will be improved.
2. Preconception counseling and intervention may occur in the context of care for other medical conditions.
3. Preconception counseling consists of three primary activities: (a) risk identification/assessment, (b) patient education, and (c) risk intervention, when possible.
4. The postpartum period is often an ideal opportunity for preconception counseling for subsequent pregnancies.

Background

Multiple independent factors impact the course and outcome of pregnancy. Figure 2.1 represents a schematic diagram of many of these factors and their interrelationship during the course of pregnancy. Prior to conception, a number of factors combine to provide the background environment in which subsequent pregnancies will develop. In particular, a complex interaction between the patient-related factors

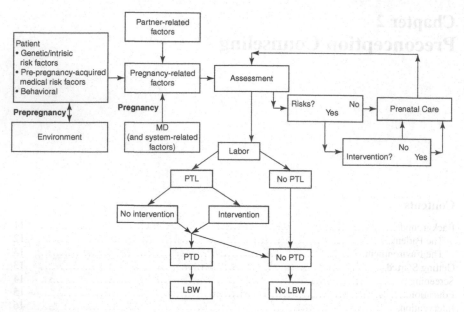

Fig. 2.1 Pregnancy outline

and environmentally related factors contributes to the likelihood of pregnancy, prenatal course, pregnancy outcomes, and postpartum complications.

The Patient

Any woman who becomes pregnant brings with her a variety of genetic and acquired factors that have the potential to impact the course of pregnancy. Genetic predisposition plays a significant role in obvious ways (e.g., sickle cell trait, Tay–Sachs, cystic fibrosis) or in more subtle manners (e.g., polymorphic tumor necrosis factor-α which may contribute to a predisposition to preterm labor). Anatomic factors may also contribute (e.g., congenital cervical incompetence, anomalous uterus). Physiological considerations such as the function of the hypothalamic–pituitary–ovarian axis (e.g., oligomenorrhea, anovulatory cycles) also play a role in becoming pregnant and in maintaining pregnancy.

Pregnancy is one potential medical event in the life of a woman, but it is by no means the only one. In addition to the genetic, anatomic, and physiological factors, many women will also acquire medical conditions that may impact the course or outcome of pregnancy. Such conditions as diabetes mellitus, hypertension, and cardiac, renal, or thyroid disease all impact the course of subsequent pregnancies. Not only do underlying disease conditions have the potential to directly impact obstetrical outcomes, many of the medications and treatments for these conditions may also have obstetrical implications. Surgical interventions involving cervical, pelvic, or intra-abdominal manipulation may also have consequences in pregnancy.

A variety of behavioral issues have direct bearing on pregnancy. Nutritional status is critical and has been the focus of recent recommended interventions such as folate supplementation prior to pregnancy. Much work has focused on the detrimental effects that tobacco, alcohol, and other drug use may have during pregnancy. Intrauterine growth rates, congenital anomalies, infant addiction, and preterm complications—among others—have all been shown to be impacted by the use of these substances. Patient exercise, fitness, and activity levels may also contribute to pregnancy outcomes.

The Environment

Although potentially less obvious, the environment in which the woman lives may contribute significantly to obstetrical outcomes. For example, lower socioeconomic status is associated with higher complication rates and/or less good outcomes in a variety of obstetrical conditions such as preterm labor, pregnancy-induced hypertension, and others. Family and partner support for the pregnancy may impact the degree to which women access care during pregnancy.

All of these factors are present prior to conception providing the biopsychosocial environment in which the pregnancy will occur. Because these factors are all present—potentially identifiable and potentially modifiable—prior to conception, it is helpful to consider pregnancy and prenatal care as beginning prior to conception as well.

Preconception counseling is a medical evaluation and intervention performed prior to conception with the expectation that the course and outcome of subsequent pregnancies will be improved. Preconception counseling offers providers an opportunity to assess, document, and potentially alter many of the factors that influence pregnancy outcome. Many patients will present to their provider only after discovering they are pregnant. Under such circumstances, the opportunity to impact this potentially critical period is lost. For this reason, preconception counseling is of paramount importance for all providers who care for women of childbearing age. Prior to pregnancy, some women will only seek care for other medical problems. Preconception counseling and intervention, therefore, may need to occur only in the context of care for other medical conditions.

Getting Started

Some women may raise the issue of planning for pregnancy providing the opportunity for the provider to begin the preconception assessment. For these women, providers can begin the process of risk identification/assessment, patient education, and risk intervention/reduction (when possible). Other women, however, may benefit from prompting by their provider. There are a number of ways in which to approach the issue, and each provider will determine for him or herself the approach that works best. Because preconception counseling will often be initiated during visits for non-obstetrical care, providers should be prepared to raise the issue in these contexts. A review of menstrual history as part of a routine exam might be followed by open-ended questioning such as "Tell me about any plans you might have to become pregnant." Visits for chronic medical conditions might lead providers to raise the issue of "the impact of this condition should you choose to become pregnant." Routine gynecological visits provide another opportunity for beginning pre-pregnancy planning. Visits related to unprotected sex (sexually transmitted disease screening, late menses, pregnancy testing, etc.) provide an excellent and natural opportunity to discuss issues of importance prior to pregnancy. An often underutilized opportunity for preconception counseling is during routine postpartum care. Planning for subsequent pregnancies (or their prevention) can begin while the patient is still in the hospital and continue when she returns for routine outpatient postpartum care.

Screening

As noted in Table 2.1, preconception counseling should include screening for issues related to the patient and to her environment (including occupational, financial, and family-related issues, among others). A variety of standardized prenatal care flow

Table 2.1 Content of preconception counseling	Patient-related factors
	Psychosocial issues
	Tobacco, alcohol, illicit drug use
	Psychiatric illness
	Literacy/language barriers
	Medications
	Prescription
	Over the counter
	Herbal, natural, and complementary/alternative therapeutics
	Medical
	Hypertension
	Obesity
	Diabetes
	Thyroid disease
	Systemic lupus erythematosus
	Renal disease
	Cardiac disease
	Thromboembolic disease
	Sickle cell disease (or trait)

Table 2.1 (Continued)

Hepatitis
HIV/AIDS
Measles (including immune status)
Varicella (including immune status)
Intra-abdominal or pelvic surgery
Obstetrics/gynecology
Pelvic anomalies
Pelvic inflammatory disease
Prior obstetrical history (all outcomes including full-term, preterm, spontaneous, and elective abortions, living children)
Macrosomic infants
Fetal/neonatal death
Genetic (patient, patient's family, and partner)
Down syndrome
Neural tube defects
Cystic fibrosis
Congenital anomalies
Multiple gestation
Environmental factors
Psychosocial issues
Physical/sexual abuse
Partner/family support
Child care
Transportation
Financial support
Insurance status
Occupational issues
High-risk occupations
Occupational exposures

sheets exist that capture much of this data. Less formal screening may be appropriate under many circumstances. For patients who are seen regularly, screening may occur sequentially over time and should be updated periodically to ensure accuracy.

Education

An appropriate preconception history will allow providers to develop a list of important pregnancy-related concerns prior to conception. This list can form the focus of ongoing education designed to allow patients to make the best possible decisions concerning their health. Modifiable risk factors can be identified and addressed as noted here. For other issues, intervention or modification may be less important than education and discussion of the identified risk factors. Providers of preconception counseling can facilitate their patients' decisions concerning the desirability and timing of and preparation for pregnancy.

Genetics counseling may be beneficial for those patients at high risk for genetic complications during pregnancy. For patients with chronic medical conditions, the risks of pregnancy, optimal timing for pregnancy, contraception (if pregnancy is medically contraindicated), and prenatal management in the case of pregnancy should all be discussed.

Counseling regarding travel should also be addressed. If a patient (or partner in some cases) has travelled, or is planning to travel to certain areas of the globe, pregnancy should potentially be delayed due to possible exposure to endemic diseases (e.g., Zika).

Intervention

A number of important interventions can be offered for women who are not yet pregnant. Patients should be counseled concerning the role of prepregnancy well-being including nutrition, exercise, and fitness. Patients should be counseled concerning the benefits of smoking cessation both for overall health and specifically related to pregnancy. Patients should be made aware of the effects of alcohol and the need to eliminate alcohol consumption prior to becoming pregnant. Use of illicit drugs should also be discouraged. Optimization of prepregnancy weight should also be addressed, and increasing BMI increases risk for many pregnancy complications for both mother and fetus.

For those patients who do not plan to become pregnant for at least 1 month, review of the vaccination history may reveal the need for administration of measles, mumps, and rubella (MMR), varicella, and hepatitis B vaccines. For patients planning to become pregnant in the near future, folic acid supplementation is recommended. For patients with known risk factors (see Table 2.1) for neural tube defects, 4 mg per day is recommended. Because fewer than half of all cases of neural tube defects occur in patients with known risk factors starting prenatal, vitamins and/or folic acid supplementation (0.4 mg per day) should be recommended for all patients prior to conception.

Patients' medical conditions and medications should be reviewed for potential complications in pregnancy. For patients who take medications contraindicated or relatively contraindicated in pregnancy, providers should discuss the risks and benefits of such medications in pregnancy. Consultation with a maternal–fetal medicine specialist may be beneficial in these circumstances.

Perhaps the single most common medical comorbidity affecting pregnancy is obesity. According to the most recent Centers for Disease Control and Prevention data, 35.7% of adults 20–39 years old are obese. As obesity is associated with many pregnancy complications including gestational diabetes and increased risk of surgical delivery, among others, it should be addressed at the preconception visit and a plan for weight loss put into place.

Ideally weight loss would occur prior to pregnancy. Weight loss prior to pregnancy can increase chances of conception and decrease rates of aforementioned pregnancy complications. If weight loss prior to conception isn't an option, then attention should be turned to appropriate weight gain during the pregnancy. Overweight women (BMI 25–29.9) should look to gain between 15 and 25 pounds over the course of their pregnancy, and obese women (BMI >/= 30) should gain no more than 11–20 pounds.

A topic related to weight is diet. At the preconception or early prenatal visit, diet should be discussed, and taking cultural/regional diet into consideration, dietary recommendations should be made. While there are many food items that can contribute to a healthy diet before and during pregnancy, some should be limited or avoided. Alcohol should be avoided during pregnancy and caffeine limited. In general long-lived predatory oceangoing fish should be limited or avoided as these accumulate mercury, which is toxic to the neurological system of the developing fetus. Deli meats, hot dogs, and unpasteurized dairy products should be avoided to decrease the risk of *L. monocytogenes* infection.

Exercise in pregnancy is largely beneficial, and unless contraindicated, women can continue pre-existing activities as tolerated in pregnancy. The amount and intensity of exercise is clearly variable based on the individual. Strenuous physical activity regimens should generally not be started during pregnancy. Occupational physical activity has limited evidence for recommendations. Most recently NIOSH proposed a guideline for lifting in pregnancy in 2013. This guideline provides provisional lifting guidelines based on gestational age, lifting activity and repetition among other criteria. While high quality evidence is lacking in this area this provisional guideline serves as a good starting place for providers and their patients.

It is also important to consider the possibility of pregnancy in patients with severe medical disease or those receiving medical therapy that is both necessary for health and contraindicated in pregnancy. The possibility of becoming pregnant should be addressed and contraception initiated in such patients.

Other issues such as language, financial, or family support barriers can be discussed, and problem-solving can begin prior to rather than after conception. Patients for whom insurance or financial issues may be an issue should be made aware of insurance programs—available in most states—to provide insurance for pregnant patients.

Chapter 3
Prenatal Care

Contents

Background... 20
Key Domains of Prenatal Information................................... 21
Frequency of Prenatal Visits... 22
   The First Prenatal Visit.. 22
   History... 22
Physical Examination.. 25
Laboratory and Diagnostic Testing....................................... 25
Estimating Gestational Age.. 26
Laboratory Testing.. 27
Treatment and Follow-Up.. 27
   Follow-Up Prenatal Visits... 27
Interval History and Physical Exam....................................... 28
   Structure of Prenatal Visits... 28
Interval Laboratory and Diagnostic Studies............................ 29

> **Key Points**
> 1. Prenatal care is a process not an event.
> 2. Excellent prenatal care represents a partnership between the provider, the patient, and her family.
> 3. Key domains of intake information in prenatal care include pregnancy dating, baseline maternal health status, family health history, medical conditions impacted by pregnancy, medical conditions impacting pregnancy, and infection.
> 4. Key domains of information during follow-up visits include normal growth and development, medical and/or obstetrical complications of pregnancy, and onset of labor.

© Springer Nature Switzerland AG 2020
P. Lyons, N. McLaughlin, *Obstetrics in Family Medicine*, Current Clinical Practice,
https://doi.org/10.1007/978-3-030-39888-0_3

Background

Prenatal care is generally the most prolonged and sustained component of pregnancy care. Such care is often delivered by a single provider who will follow the course of the pregnancy with nearly as much interest as the pregnant patient. Although the prenatal period is often filled with anxiety, it is generally more relaxed and almost always less pressured than the labor and delivery setting. For these reasons, prenatal care provides patients with an opportunity to educate themselves and participate in the process of preparing for a new infant.

Prenatal care can best be thought of as a process rather than a specific event. For patients who received preconception counseling, it is a continuation of the threefold process of education, risk identification, and risk reduction/intervention. For those patients who did not receive preconception counseling, it should be the beginning of such a process. Many prenatal care providers also participate in the delivery of their patients. In this regard, prenatal care provides an opportunity to establish or enhance a relationship that stretches from preconception through prenatal management to delivery. Excellent prenatal care represents a partnership between the provider and the pregnant patient (and her family) with ample opportunity for discussion, questions, and answers and active participation by each person involved.

Prenatal care is a cornerstone of modern obstetric care and has accompanied a reduction in the historic risk associated with pregnancy. Maternal mortality in 1935 was 582 per 100,000 pregnancies. By 1993, that figure had decreased to 7.5 per 100,000. Over approximately the same period, infant mortality decreased from 47 per 1000 to 8 per 100,000. Although many factors unrelated to prenatal care have contributed to these reductions, prenatal care has directly contributed to improved outcomes in a variety of areas: (a) fetal organogenesis (folic acid supplementation, glycemic control in diabetes), (b) infectious disease detection/treatment (e.g., chlamydia, bacteriuria), (c) infectious disease transmission prevention (e.g., syphilis, HIV), and (d) fetal growth (e.g., glycemic control in gestational diabetes).

Figure 2.1 in Chap. 2 provides a schematic outline for the interrelated factors involved in pregnancy. Factors present during the preconception period were reviewed in the prior chapter. With the advent of conception, additional factors come into play. Pregnancy itself introduces a variety of new conditions that can impact the health of both the mother and the infant. Although less well described, a variety of paternal factors can also affect the course and outcome of pregnancy. Although not specifically addressed in this chapter, there are a number of physician- and system-related factors that can, likewise, impact pregnancy. The process of prenatal care is cyclical and repetitive. Each visit allows providers to review what has already happened and to determine what has developed in the interval since the last visit. Each visit will focus on patient education, determination of normal growth and development, and compilation of critical information in a variety of important domains.

Key Domains of Prenatal Information

The first step in any prenatal assessment is to confirm that the patient is, in fact, pregnant. Many patients will arrive for a first prenatal visit with a confirmed positive pregnancy test result. Other patients will arrive for their first "prenatal" visit with a variety of less clear presentations. They may have missed their period but not have been tested. They may have self-tested but not trust the results (either positive or negative). Regardless of the nature of the uncertainty, all patients with uncertain pregnancy status should have their status confirmed via urine or serum human chorionic gonadotropin (hCG) testing. Following confirmation of pregnancy, all patients should have the opportunity to consider what the most appropriate next step should be. When uncertain regarding the desirability of a confirmed pregnancy, providers should be cautious in their choice of language. In particular, providers should avoid the use of language that implies a specific outcome such as "Congratulations, you're pregnant!" or "We will need to get you started with prenatal care soon." The use of open-ended questions such as "The test confirms that you are pregnant. How do you feel about that?" will allow patients to more easily express their thoughts concerning subsequent management. In any patient who was not planning on becoming pregnant, options counseling should be provided, using specific non-leading language. As with any situation in medicine, a patient can only make an informed decision when all options are understood.

Initial evaluation during prenatal care is similar to the evaluation for preconception counseling. It is designed to focus on the patient's baseline condition and any development in the time frame from the last menstrual period (LMP) through the first prenatal visit. (This is a time period during which patients may not recognize that they are pregnant and may include significant exposures to infectious or toxic agents.) At intake prenatal screening provides important information in six key domains:

1. Baseline maternal health including prior obstetrical history, if any
2. Family health (e.g., twins, Down syndrome, Tay–Sachs)
3. Medical conditions impacted by pregnancy (e.g., cardiac disease, renal disease)
4. Medical conditions impacting pregnancy (e.g., diabetes mellitus, hypertension, medications, toxic exposures)
5. Infection
6. Pregnancy dating

As discussed in the previous chapter, these domains of information can form the basis for patient education and intervention throughout the course of pregnancy (and beyond).

Following the initial prenatal screen, subsequent visits focus on interval developments and review of previously identified issues. It is often helpful to develop a prenatal problem list to organize ongoing issues under management. Such a list could include the problem; the date identified; interventions, if any; and the date resolved, if applicable. Follow-up prenatal care will focus on three key domains: (a) normal growth and development, (b) medical and/or obstetrical complications of pregnancy, and (c) onset of labor.

Frequency of Prenatal Visits

The frequency of visits during prenatal care is dependent on the complexity of the care being provided. For those patients with complex presentations, individualized decisions must be made concerning the frequency of prenatal visits. For patients with uncomplicated pregnancies, the currently recommended frequency for visits is as follows:

- First prenatal visit: in the first trimester
- Follow-up visits: every 4 weeks until 30 weeks of gestation, then every 2 weeks until 36 weeks of gestation, then every week until delivery at term, or twice weekly from 40 weeks for assessment of fetal well-being (see Chap. 18)

The First Prenatal Visit (See Table 3.1)

The first prenatal visit lays the groundwork for all subsequent visits and therefore includes the most comprehensive history, physical examination, and diagnostic testing. For patients who have had one or more preconception counseling visits, much of the information can be obtained from the records of those visits. Information subject to change will need to be updated, and a brief review of all material should be performed to ensure accuracy and completeness. Many offices utilize one of the many standardized obstetrical health history and prenatal flow sheet forms that exist in both paper and electronic form. In addition to providing a standardized method for recording necessary information, the flow sheets can serve as a prompt for providers throughout the course of pregnancy.

History

Menstrual History The preconception history begins with the LMP. Information should include the date of the first day of bleeding and the duration. The certainty of this date is of considerable importance as this forms the first basis for predicting the estimated date of delivery (EDD, or confinement in some older references). Depending on a variety of factors, including regularity of menses, duration since LMP, and whether patients track menses regularly, patient's recall of their LMP may be of variable reliability. Some notation of the patient's subjective "certainty" con-

Table 3.1 First prenatal visit

Last menstrual period (LMP)
Duration, abnormalities, fertility treatment, contraceptive use, and prior pregnancies
Prior obstetrical history: all prior pregnancies including elective and spontaneous abortions
All pregnancies: date, outcome, weeks of gestation
Deliveries: gender and weight of infant, duration of labor, delivery method, anesthesia, and complications, if any
General medical history: including all pertinent medical conditions but focused on:
Anesthesia history
Medications
Medication allergies
Toxic exposures (including tobacco, alcohol, and illicit drugs)
History since LMP: events or exposures during early organogenesis
Drugs, medications, and radiation
Infectious diseases (cytomegalovirus, toxoplasmosis, tuberculosis)
Possible pregnancy-related symptoms (bleeding or discharge per vagina, abdominal pain, headache, visual complaints, emesis)
Family history: comprehensive but with an emphasis on:
Fetal deaths or abnormalities
Multiple gestations
Genetic history (cystic fibrosis, Down syndrome, thalassemia)
Chronic medical conditions with strong familial link (e.g., hypertension, diabetes mellitus, renal disease, substance abuse)
Safety
Abuse, including sexual abuse
Domestic violence
Seat belt use
Environmental risks including work-related hazards

cerning the date should be recorded. First-trimester bleeding is a relatively common complaint and may mimic menstruation. For this reason, patients should be questioned concerning the timing and quantity of bleeding as well. A "period" that is abnormally light or heavy or fell out of the normal cycle may represent an event of pregnancy rather than the true LMP.

Prior Obstetrical History Prior obstetrical history can significantly impact the current pregnancy. For this reason all prior pregnancies should be summarized in the prenatal record. For all prior pregnancies, documentation should include the date of the pregnancy, the outcome (full-term delivery, preterm delivery, spontaneous abortion, elective abortion), and the weeks of gestation completed. For those pregnancies that resulted in live delivery, additional key information would include date of delivery, gender and weight of the infant, duration of labor, delivery method and anesthesia use, or complications, if any.

This information can be summarized in shorthand form as gravida/para figures. This notation takes the form of G_xP_{xxxx}. G(ravida) represents the total number of pregnancies regardless of outcome. P(ara) represents, in order from left to right, full-term deliveries, preterm deliveries, abortions (elective or spontaneous), and living children. Although it does not include all of the details of each pregnancy, this shorthand form provides a quick and convenient summary that is especially useful in oral or written presentations.

General Medical History All pregnancies occur within the context of the patient's baseline health status. Many medical conditions may impact the course of pregnancy. At the same time, pregnancy may have a significant effect on a variety of pre-existing medical conditions. It should also be recognized that delivery is a surgical procedure in many instances with approximately one-fourth of all deliveries occurring via cesarean section. For this reason, a comprehensive review of the patient's general medical history should be recorded. Special emphasis should be placed on chronic medical conditions, prior surgical and anesthesia history, medications, medication allergies, and substance use including tobacco, alcohol, and illicit drug use. In addition, chronic back pain or spinal conditions are often relevant history for the pregnant patient as neuraxial anesthesia (spinal or epidural) is the most common form of labor analgesia and its availability to the patient can be impacted by these conditions. If questions occur a pre-labor consultation with anesthesia can greatly clarify pain relief options for a specific patient.

History Since LMP Particular attention should be paid to medical events between the LMP and the first prenatal period. This represents the critical period of organogenesis during which a variety of medical conditions and exposures may have a significant impact on the developing fetus. In particular, note should be made concerning management and/or control of chronic medical conditions that may impact fetal development such as hypertension and diabetes mellitus. Exposure to a variety of toxic and infectious agents is also important during this time period. Note should be made of exposure to drugs, medications, live vaccine preparations, or radiation. Known or suspected exposure to infectious agents should also be documented including travel to endemic areas, sexually transmitted disease, cytomegalovirus, toxoplasmosis, tuberculosis, HIV, rubella, or varicella.

In addition to exposures, this period of early pregnancy is also marked by a variety of potential complications of pregnancy such as abnormal implantation or hyperemesis gravidarum. Patients should be screened for possible pregnancy-related symptoms such as bleeding or abnormal discharge per vagina, abdominal pain, headache, visual complaints, and severe nausea or vomiting.

Family History A number of familial conditions and events are of potential consequence in pregnancy. A family history should be obtained with an emphasis on fetal deaths or abnormalities, multiple gestations, gestational diabetes, large- or small-for-gestational-age infants, significant genetic history (e.g., cystic fibrosis, Down syndrome, thalassemia), and chronic medical conditions with a strong familial link such as hypertension, diabetes, renal disease, and substance abuse.

Physical Examination

All patients should receive a comprehensive physical examination. The purpose of the examination is threefold:

1. Diagnostic or supportive evidence of underlying medical conditions
2. Notation of normal physical changes often associated with pregnancy
3. Evaluation of the uterus and bony pelvis

A variety of physical changes can be noted during pregnancy. Although underlying medical conditions must be excluded, these findings generally represent benign changes and should be noted primarily for reference in case of change. Such findings include split S1 and/or a systolic ejection murmur on cardiac examination, mild thyroid enlargement, skin changes including malar rash and striae gravidarum, and accentuated lordosis noted on musculoskeletal examination.

Evaluation of uterine size is helpful in confirming the gestational age. At 6 weeks' gestation, the uterus has enlarged beyond its prepregnant dimensions and is described as the size of an orange. By 8–10 weeks, the uterus is described as grapefruit sized. At 10–12 weeks, the uterus is palpable on abdominal examination at the symphysis pubis. Once the uterus is palpable from the abdomen, measurement is made of the fundal height. This measurement represents the distance from the symphysis pubis to the top of the uterine fundus. By 20 weeks' gestation, the uterine fundus should normally be found at the level of the umbilicus. From 20 to 34 weeks' gestation, measurement of the fundal height (in cm) should be equivalent to the gestational age (in weeks). For example, at 28 weeks' gestation, the fundal height should be approximately 28 cm from symphysis to the top of the uterine fundus (±2 cm). Any significant deviation from these expected measurements should prompt the provider to reassess the gestational age and/or fetal development.

Assessment of the bony pelvic configuration (clinical pelvimetry) is often performed early in pregnancy to determine potential structural impediments to successful delivery. Abnormal findings do not rule out the possibility of a trial of labor and successful vaginal delivery, but added caution may be warranted at the time of delivery. Notation should be made of the diagonal conjugate (distance from symphysis pubis to sacral promontory), ischial spines (blunt, prominent), sacrum (concave, straight), coccyx (fixed, mobile), and pubic arch (normal, wide, narrow).

Laboratory and Diagnostic Testing

As previously noted, all patients for whom pregnancy status is uncertain should have a confirmatory pregnancy test. This may take the form of either a urine or serum test for hCG. The urine hCG test is generally positive beginning at the time of the first missed period (approximately 4 weeks' gestation). The serum test is generally positive at the time of implantation.

For all prenatal patients, routine obstetrical laboratory screening should include complete blood count with platelets, blood type (ABO and Rh), rapid plasma reagin, rubella titer, hepatitis B surface antigen (to detect active disease), HIV antibody, Papanicolaou smear (if not performed within the preceding 3 months), gonorrhea and chlamydia screen, and routine urine analysis with culture.

Selected patients may also benefit from screening for the following conditions: sickle cell disease (via routine screen or hemoglobin electrophoresis), Tay–Sachs, toxoplasmosis, cytomegalovirus, elevated serum lead, elevated glucose, substance use, and/or herpes simplex virus.

These screening tests are recommended at the first prenatal visit, which should routinely occur in the first trimester. For those patients who present for a first prenatal visit later in pregnancy, laboratory and diagnostic testing should include those tests just mentioned as well as all tests appropriate to their estimated gestational age at the time of presentation. These additional tests are described later.

Estimating Gestational Age

At the conclusion of the first prenatal visit, a clinical assessment of gestational age and estimated date of delivery should be established. If the available information is incomplete or contradictory, a tentative date may be assigned with arrangements for acquisition of more definitive data.

The available data that may contribute to the establishment of the gestational age includes the following:

1. LMP: if the menstrual history is certain, an accurate calculation can be made based on the first day of the LMP. Obstetrical calendars (often referred to as an "OB wheel") are available (both physical and electronic, online or as an app for smartphones) that allow such calculation. In the absence of such a wheel, the EDD can be calculated by subtracting 3 months and adding 1 week to the LMP. For example, if the first day of the LMP was April 14, subtracting 3 months would yield January 14 and adding 1 week would then yield January 21 of the following year as the EDD.
2. Physical examination: as noted previously, uterine size can be used to give a clinical estimate of gestational age. When this data is congruent with the LMP, it is generally accurate to within 1 week.
3. Developmental milestones: the fetal heartbeat should be detectable with a hand-held Doppler at approximately 10 weeks of gestation and with a fetoscope at 18–20 weeks. Fetal quickening (fetal movement) should be reported by the mother at 18–20 weeks' gestation.
4. Ultrasound: an obstetric ultrasound obtained early in pregnancy (first trimester or early second trimester) is accurate to within approximately 1 week of gestation. The accuracy of ultrasound dating diminishes with advancing fetal age. In

the third trimester, fetal ultrasound is accurate to within 2 weeks up to 36 weeks' gestation and within 3 weeks thereafter. For full breakdown of ultrasound dating, the American College of Obstetrics and Gynecology (ACOG) guidelines on ultrasound dating provide an excellent reference.

Laboratory Testing

Levels of hCG obtained via quantitative testing are not considered accurate for dating purposes as significant variability is noted at any given gestational age.

As a general rule, the first gestational age/EDD assigned should remain unchanged throughout the pregnancy unless significant doubt exists concerning the data used to establish that date. Caution should be exercised when "correcting" an EDD based on later data.

Treatment and Follow-Up

All patients who are planning on continuing with their pregnancy and not already taking prenatal vitamins should be given a prescription and encouraged to immediately begin taking one vitamin per day. In addition, iron supplementation should be considered for those patients with documented anemia.

At the first prenatal visit, patients should be given an overview of the course of prenatal care, a general caution concerning warning symptoms that should prompt early follow-up, and arrangements should be made for an appropriate follow-up visit. Patients should be given the opportunity to ask questions and to clarify any areas of uncertainty. It may be helpful to suggest that patients keep a list of written questions between visits to help ensure that all important concerns are addressed at each visit.

Follow-Up Prenatal Visits

Follow-up visits are designed to meet four purposes: to track the progress of the pregnancy; early identification of complications, if any; completion of testing/evaluation at specific gestational-age milestones; and patient education/anticipatory guidance.

Follow-up visits provide the opportunity to elicit patient questions and concerns and to provide education and counseling. Topics for review include nutritional status, activity and exercise in pregnancy, and symptoms consistent with preterm labor.

Plans for delivery, such as when to contact the provider and when to go to the hospital, should be addressed. Also discussed should be issues related to delivery and the postpartum period, including use of anesthesia, breastfeeding, circumcision, and the duration of the postpartum stay.

Follow-up intervals noted here are for uncomplicated pregnancies. Follow-up must be arranged as indicated should abnormalities present at any point.

Interval History and Physical Exam

Structure of Prenatal Visits

In the absence of complications or extenuating circumstances, prenatal visits will fall into a general pattern that roughly fits by trimester. Given that prenatal visits occur across a prolonged period, each visit itself is brief and to the point. The interval history should focus primarily on events and developments in the time period from the last visit to the current visit. Review of unresolved or ongoing concerns should also occur. Aspects of the history that should be addressed at every visit would include fetal movement (presence or absence and quantity), uterine contractions, pelvic pain or pressure, abdominal or back pain, and discharge or bleeding per vagina.

First Trimester

Visits in the first trimester will be focused on establishing medical history and physical norms for the patient. Visits in this trimester are the least frequent, occurring once every 4 weeks. Mainly the visit will focus on answering patient questions, providing education, treating the symptoms of early pregnancy, and obtaining genetic screening and dating exams as appropriate. Educational goals should be around setting patient expectations for pregnancy. Early education about breastfeeding should be initiated as it has been shown to increase breastfeeding rates and women have often made their decision on whether or not to breast feed by the third trimester.

Second Trimester

During second trimester visits, the fetus is assessed with surveillance tests, maternal weight gain is monitored, and education about expected and unexpected pregnancy events and complications is discussed.

Third Trimester

Third trimester visits will have the clinician check a few last screening tests, monitoring of mother and fetus will continue, and education will shift toward the labor and delivery and postpartum course with discussions of postdelivery contraception and topics such as early parenting.

The physical examination contributes to assessment of fetal development and may also provide clues to the detection of pregnancy-related complications. The core elements of the physical examination include blood pressure, notation of edema, and weight. Assessments of fetal development include measurement of fundal height and documentation of the fetal heart rate.

Appropriate weight gain in pregnancy is a very common concern for pregnant patients. In population studies, optimal outcomes have been associated with maternal weight gain of 20–25 lb. during pregnancy. Current recommendations for weight gain during pregnancy suggest 25–35 lb. for a woman of average weight at the onset of pregnancy. Decreased weight gain can be associated with inadequate nutritional intake, inaccurate dating, intrauterine growth retardation, oligohydramnios, and fetal demise. Increased weight gain can be associated with excessive caloric intake, inaccurate dating, macrosomia, multiple gestation, and polyhydramnios. Abnormal weight gain should prompt review of the prenatal course, eating patterns, and fetal well-being surveillance.

Interval Laboratory and Diagnostic Studies

Each pregnancy will require individualization of appropriate interval laboratory and diagnostic studies. For most pregnancies, however, a variety of interval studies should be considered:

1. At 11–14 weeks' gestation, screening for chromosomal abnormalities can be performed as mentioned in Chap. 6.
2. At 15–20 weeks' gestation, patients not screened earlier should be offered maternal triple (hCG, alpha fetal protein, and estriol) or quadruple (hCG, alpha fetal protein, estriol, inhibin) screening for developmental abnormalities. In addition, an obstetrical ultrasound is often ordered in this time period although it may be ordered earlier or later for specific indications. At 24–28 weeks' gestation, patients should undergo glucose challenge testing for gestational diabetes, repeat hemoglobin (28 weeks), and antibody screen (28 weeks).
3. At 35–37 weeks, RPR, Hep B sAg, HIV, GC/chlamydia, and group B strep are all indicated.

Chapter 4
Medications in Pregnancy

Contents

Background.. 32
General Principles of Medication Use in Pregnancy........................... 32
   Chronic Medical Conditions.. 32
   Acute Medical Conditions.. 33
   Acute Obstetrical Conditions.. 34
   Therapeutic Categories and Considerations................................. 34
Proven Human Teratogens.. 35
Special Considerations.. 36
   Tobacco.. 36
   Alcohol... 37
   Illicit Drugs... 37
Over-the-Counter Medications... 37
   OTC Pain Medications... 38
Acetaminophen... 38
Aspirin.. 38
Nonsteroidal Anti-inflammatory Drugs.. 39
   OTC Cough/Cold/Allergy Medications....................................... 39
Antihistamines... 39
Decongestants.. 39
Cough Medications.. 40

Key Points
1. All medications should be viewed with caution in pregnancy.
2. Management of medication use in pregnancy ideally begins with adequate preconception counseling and prepregnancy planning.
3. Medications used in pregnancy require clear identification of indication for use, duration of treatment, expected outcome, and signs or symptoms requiring early termination of their use.
4. When in doubt consultation with an expert in maternal–fetal medicine is strongly recommended.

© Springer Nature Switzerland AG 2020
P. Lyons, N. McLaughlin, *Obstetrics in Family Medicine*, Current Clinical Practice,
https://doi.org/10.1007/978-3-030-39888-0_4

Background

With the exception of prenatal vitamins and possibly iron supplementation, all medications should be used with caution during pregnancy. Although clinical experience with many medications in pregnancy is quite extensive and the safety and efficacy are reasonably established, pregnancy represents a unique challenge in medication assessment. It would not be ethical, under most circumstances, to randomize pregnant patients to receive increasing doses of medications to assess safety and efficacy of a medication known to produce or suspected of producing harm in pregnancy. This limits the degree to which safety can be categorically stated for the use of any medication in pregnancy. Many medications once thought to be safe in pregnancy have subsequently been shown to be harmful. Other medications originally thought to be harmful have been shown to have beneficial effects when used for specific medically indicated purposes.

Many medications can and should be used in pregnancy for a variety of legitimate medical indications. Although it is beyond the scope of this chapter to discuss in detail the use of all medications in pregnancy, a few general guidelines can be offered. Texts exist that detail the risks and benefits of many available medications. Such a text should be a routine part of every obstetrical provider's library. When doubt exists concerning the indications for or the safety or efficacy of any medication, consultation with an expert in maternal–fetal medicine is strongly recommended.

General Principles of Medication Use in Pregnancy

The three general principles are as follows:

1. Chronic medications should be reviewed to assess safety and efficacy.
2. The risk of not treating (or treating less effectively) an identified disease (acute or chronic) should be weighed against the risks of the proposed treatment.
3. All medications used in pregnancy require clear identification of indication for use, duration of treatment, expected outcomes, and signs or symptoms that require early termination of use.

Chronic Medical Conditions

Some patients have chronic medical conditions that predate pregnancy. The management of many of these conditions will include the use of medication. Although it is always important to consider safety and efficacy when using medications, with the onset of pregnancy, these considerations become considerably more complex. Ideally, a consideration of the impact of pregnancy on the medical condition as well as the impact of the medical condition on pregnancy would occur prior to pregnancy. For some patients, this leads to a recommendation to delay pregnancy until the medical condition can be more adequately controlled. In other circumstances, it may lead to a recommendation to avoid pregnancy altogether.

Under many circumstances (both planned and unplanned), however, management of pregnancy will overlap with management of chronic medical conditions and their associated medications. The first consideration should be for the safety of the mother. Disease processes that are life-threatening to the mother may require continuation of treatment even if pregnancy is continued. The provider should explore treatment alternatives with equal efficacy and better established safety profiles when possible. When safer alternatives are not available, providers should discuss with patients the potential risks of continuing the pregnancy while simultaneously continuing the use of the required medication versus the potential risks of terminating medication use for the duration of pregnancy. Patients must be given sufficient information to make an informed decision concerning their health and the health of their developing fetus, especially during the critical period of organogenesis early in pregnancy. In all circumstances, providers and patients must make individualized treatment decisions based on the medical conditions of the specific patient.

Acute Medical Conditions

Pregnant patients are vulnerable to all the acute medical conditions of nonpregnant patients. Medical decisions concerning the treatment of acute medical conditions that arise during pregnancy must follow the same general guidelines as those for chronic conditions. Will the medical condition adversely affect the pregnancy? Will treatment of the condition ameliorate or eliminate these potential effects? Will the proposed treatment adversely affect the pregnancy? Are there safer or more well-established alternative treatment options? What are the *likely* consequences of not treating the medical condition? What are the *potential* consequences of not treating the medical condition?

As with the treatment of chronic medical conditions, it is critical that both providers and patients have sufficient information concerning the risks and benefits of treatment options to make informed, individualized decisions. When providers cannot adequately answer these questions, patients should be referred to a provider with sufficient expertise to provide more complete information.

Acute Obstetrical Conditions

Pregnancy may be accompanied by a variety of complications that require consideration of medication use. The same general principles apply, and the same questions must be answered. When these complications are relatively common, much established data may exist to guide providers and patients in their decision-making process. When the complications are less common, consultation may be required.

Therapeutic Categories and Considerations

Any drug used during pregnancy should be checked for safety prior to use. Keeping in mind the general considerations just given, the following recommendations may be considered:

1. When antibiotics are indicated consider penicillin, cephalosporins (except cefotetan), clindamycin, and macrolides. Avoid sulfa drugs (contraindicated in the first and third trimester), quinolones, tetracyclines, and aminoglycosides (ototoxic, may be indicated for severe Gram-negative infections).
2. When analgesics are indicated, consider acetaminophen and narcotic analgesia (consult reference for specific agents). Narcotic analgesics do cross the placenta and may affect the fetus transiently. Long-term narcotic analgesia use (or abuse) during pregnancy can be associated with withdrawal symptoms in the newborn. Narcotic analgesia at or near delivery has been associated with respiratory depression in newborns, which can be reversed, if necessary, with Narcan. Avoid aspirin (in analgesic doses) and nonsteroidal anti-inflammatory drugs (NSAIDs, contraindicated in late pregnancy).
3. For treatment of hypertension, consider labetalol (individual β-blockers should be reviewed prior to use as some β-blockers have been associated with adverse effects on uteroplacental and fetal hemodynamics and fetal growth), methyldopa, and hydralazine. Avoid angiotensin-converting enzymes (and angiotensin receptor blockade agents).
4. For patients with diabetes, consider insulin and regular- and intermediate-acting agents, but avoid oral hypoglycemics (recent data suggests that some oral hypoglycemics may be safely used in pregnancy, but experience is limited and individual agents should be reviewed prior to use).
5. For patients suffering from nausea, consider using Diclectin (doxylamine/pyridoxine) or chlorpromazine.
6. In cases of gastritis/peptic ulcer disease, consider magnesium hydroxide, aluminum hydroxide, calcium carbonate, and bismuth subsalicylate.

Proven Human Teratogens

Some agents have proven teratogenic potential. These agents are summarized in Table 4.1. Although the effects of such agents are potentially variable and predictable, their use should be very limited or avoided during pregnancy. Category D agents have proven teratogenic potential but may, under certain circumstances, be indicated. Prior to using any category D agent, providers should perform a careful review of indications, duration of therapy, all potential effects, and all potential alternatives to the proposed therapy. In addition, patients should be informed of these considerations, allowing for informed consent to the proposed therapy. Category X medications have proven teratogenic potential, and use should be avoided in pregnancy.

Teratogenicity is a multifactorial outcome that is related to several factors including (1) the teratogenic potential of the agent, (2) the susceptibility of the fetus, (3) the dose/duration of exposure, and (4) the timing of the exposure. As noted in Table 4.2, medications can be classified by their observed correlation with fetal harm in animal or human studies. Susceptibility may be based on the genetic factors

Table 4.1 Selected proven human teratogens	Category D
	ACE inhibitors/ARB
	Cyclophosphamide
	Lithium
	Paramethadione
	Phenytoin
	Barbiturates
	Carbamazepine
	Benzodiazepines
	Systemic retinoids
	Tetracycline
	Tamoxifen
	Trimethadione
	Valproic acid
	Warfarin
	Category X
	Thalidomide
	Methotrexate
	Danazol
	Misoprostol
	Diethylstilbestrol

Table 4.2 Medication safety ratings in pregnancy

Category A: controlled human studies have demonstrated no increased risk of fetal harm
Category B: no controlled human studies suggest increased risk; probably safe in pregnancy when use is indicated
Category C: no evidence in human studies of increased risk, but animal studies show possible increased risk
Category D: evidence in human studies suggest increased risk, but benefits of treatment may outweigh risk
Category X: clear evidence of teratogenic effects exists; contraindicated in pregnancy

as well as the gestational age of the fetus. As a general rule, very early exposure (approximately first 2 weeks of gestation) results in an all-or-none phenomenon which may result in fetal demise. Exposure during the period of organogenesis (approximately weeks 3–9) is more likely to result in major morphologic abnormalities. Exposure thereafter may result in variable defects. Although this may serve as a guideline, careful assessment and possible consultation should be considered for any patient with a significant antenatal exposure.

Special Considerations

In addition to the use of medications in pregnancy, a variety of other exposures may occur with possible effects on pregnancy. These might include occupational exposures, legal and illegal drugs, or nonpharmacological items such as exercising, lifting, or other activities. As previously noted, most such exposures will be subject to limited data concerning possible pregnancy effects. For this reason, the same general principles should apply that apply to medication use:

1. Is there any data available to guide the decision?
2. Is there a specific and compelling reason for the exposure?
3. Do safer alternatives exist?
4. Can potential adverse effects be monitored?
5. Can exposure be limited or modified in such a way as to minimize potential risks?

Although a full discussion of all such exposures is the work of an entire text in its own right, three common and frequently encountered exposures deserve attention.

Tobacco

Tobacco is associated with a variety of adverse outcomes including low birth weight, increased risk of fetal demise, abruptio placentae, and placenta previa. Although the absolute risk associated with tobacco use is not clearly defined, the outcomes are potentially quite severe. As tobacco has no known benefits in pregnancy, every effort should be made to reduce or eliminate tobacco exposure during pregnancy.

Alcohol

Fetal alcohol syndrome (FAS) is a constellation of developmental and physical findings in neonates born to mothers who consumed large quantities of alcohol during pregnancy. FAS is associated with growth retardation, microcephaly, microphthalmia, and central nervous system deficiencies. The use of alcohol is quite prevalent, and a significant number of pregnant mothers will have consumed alcohol prior to becoming pregnant. The question frequently arises whether alcohol can be safely used in any quantity during pregnancy. Although data is limited, there is no established safe level of alcohol use in pregnancy. For this reason, patients should be encouraged to eliminate or significantly limit alcohol use during pregnancy.

Illicit Drugs

A variety of illicit drugs are associated with adverse pregnancy outcomes. Each drug should be reviewed individually for specific concerns. In addition to the medical considerations, all such drugs are, by definition, illegal and carry with them significant social risk. All pregnant patients should be screened by history for illicit drug use and, when present, counseled concerning the desirability of reduction or elimination. This screening and counseling should be approached in a nonjudgmental and nonthreatening manner. A threatening or legalistic approach to patients is likely to reduce patient reporting and therefore limit providers' ability to effectively intervene.

Over-the-Counter Medications

Questions concerning the use of over-the-counter (OTC) medications arise frequently during the course of pregnancy. The general considerations for use are the same as for prescription medications. The ease of access combined with the frequency with which OTC medications are used makes recommendations in pregnancy particularly challenging. It is estimated that more than half of all medication use in the United States is OTC. Approximately 75% of all pregnant patients will use one or more OTC medication during the course of pregnancy.

Although providers can control access to prescription medications, OTC medications are, by definition, available to patients without the necessity of a prescription. In addition, the safety of OTC medications may vary with the time in pregnancy when they are used. For example, OTC NSAIDs that may be safely used early in pregnancy are generally contraindicated in the third trimester. For this reason, providers must be able to discuss in detail the appropriate uses and precautions that patients must keep in mind when deciding whether to use OTC medications during pregnancy.

Food and Drug Administration (FDA) pregnancy safety ratings are available for all OTC medications and should be reviewed prior to their use. It should be noted that supplements such as herbal and/or natural preparations are not subject. FDA oversight and information concerning safety in pregnancy may be very limited. The breadth of OTC medications available make a comprehensive review beyond the scope of this text; however, two common categories of medications warrant consideration: pain medications and cough/cold/allergy medications.

OTC Pain Medications

Pain is among the most common of medical complaints, and although the frequency of pain in pregnancy may not be higher than in the nonpregnant state, it is certainly not any less common. For this reason, patients will often seek advice from their providers on OTC pain medication options.

Acetaminophen

Acetaminophen is widely used in pregnancy and early childhood. Although randomized, controlled trials concerning the safety of acetaminophen in pregnancy are lacking, the extensive experience combined with few reports of complications makes the use of acetaminophen a safe choice in pregnancy. Acetaminophen is a category B drug in all stages of pregnancy.

Aspirin

Use of aspirin has been associated with a variety of potential pregnancy complications, including prolonged gestation and decreased birth weight. In addition, aspirin has potent antiplatelet activity that may predispose patients to bleeding. The use of aspirin in pregnancy has been associated with neonatal hemorrhage. Aspirin is a category D drug in all stages of pregnancy, and its use as an OTC medication should be discouraged during pregnancy. This is in regards to OTC aspirin used at analgesic doses. Baby aspirin (81mg) is used for a variety of pregnancy complications such as pre-eclampsia and is discussed in Chap. 15.

Nonsteroidal Anti-inflammatory Drugs

Although NSAIDs are often combined as a single class, significant differences may exist in their use during pregnancy. Indomethacin (a prescription NSAID) has been used in pregnancy for preterm labor (see Chap. 7) but has been associated with significant complications and should only be used with caution and for specific indications. OTC NSAIDs, including ibuprofen and naproxen, are category B drugs in early pregnancy but category D drugs in the third trimester. In the absence of a compelling indication for the use of NSAIDs in pregnancy, their use as an OTC medication should probably be limited.

OTC Cough/Cold/Allergy Medications

Given the duration of pregnancy, the likelihood of experiencing symptoms of allergies or viral respiratory infections is quite high. A wide variety of OTC medications are available to treat the various symptoms of viral respiratory infections and allergies, and their use is quite common in pregnancy.

Antihistamines

Chlorpheniramine is a commonly used antihistamine in a variety of allergy and cold formulations. Chlorpheniramine is a category B drug and is probably safe for use during pregnancy. Diphenhydramine is the second commonly used antihistamine and is also a category B medication. It should, however, be used with caution as it has been shown to cross the placenta, may have oxytocin-like effects at high doses, and may interact with other drugs in pregnancy.

Decongestants

Pseudoephedrine has been the subject of animal studies and has had widespread human use in pregnancy. Pseudoephedrine is a category B medication, and its use in pregnancy is probably safe. Because it has been associated with a possible increase in the risk of gastroschisis, its use in the first trimester of pregnancy should probably be avoided when possible.

Cough Medications

Cough medications fall into two broad categories: antitussive medications and expectorants. Both categories of medication are available in a wide variety of OTC formulations. Guaifenesin, a common expectorant, is a category C drug. Its use in the first trimester of pregnancy has been associated with a possible increased risk of neural tube defects, but data is limited. It is probably safest to avoid the use of guaifenesin in the first trimester of pregnancy when possible. Dextromethorphan is also a category C drug. Animal studies have shown an association between dextromethorphan exposure and birth defects. Human data has not found a similar association.

Chapter 5
Vaccines in Pregnancy

Contents

Background.. 41
Infectious Diseases in Pregnancy.. 42
Vaccines Recommended in All Pregnancies.. 42
   Influenza.. 42
   Tetanus, Diphtheria, and Pertussis (Tdap)... 43
Vaccines to Be Considered Based on Risk vs. Benefit............................... 43
   Hepatitis A... 43
   Yellow Fever... 43
   Meningococcal (B)... 43
Vaccines for Use if Indicated... 44
Vaccines Contraindicated in Pregnancy... 44

Key Points

1. Recognize that pregnant women are at an increased risk from many communicable diseases.
2. Vaccines in pregnancy can play a role in decreasing maternal risk from infectious causes.
3. There are two vaccines recommended for all pregnant patients, influenza and Tdap

---

Background

The subject of vaccines in pregnancy can be a cause for concern in both the pregnant patient and the obstetrical provider. Just as with medications, or any other intervention in pregnancy, risks and benefits should be weighed. In recent years, even the CDC has changed vaccine recommendations in pregnancy. A categorized

---

© Springer Nature Switzerland AG 2020

P. Lyons, N. McLaughlin, *Obstetrics in Family Medicine*, Current Clinical Practice,
https://doi.org/10.1007/978-3-030-39888-0_5

Table 5.1 Vaccine recommendations in pregnancy

Vaccines recommended in all pregnancies	Vaccines to be considered based on risk vs. benefit	Vaccines for use if indicated	Vaccines contraindicated in pregnancy
Influenza Tdap	Hepatitis A Yellow fever Meningococcal B	Meningococcal (ACWY) Polio Td Anthrax Rabies Smallpox	MMR Varicella Zoster

table summarizing these recommendations is present at the beginning of this chapter (Table 5.1). For screening for illness or history of vaccination of measles or varicella, please see Chap. 3.

Infectious Diseases in Pregnancy

Pregnant patients are at an increased risk from many different infections. Some infections are prevented by avoidance of certain foods or household chores, while other infections are prevented through the administration of appropriate vaccinations. Below is a brief discussion of the different vaccines that could be used during pregnancy according to risk factors of the specific patient and also of vaccines that should be avoided during pregnancy. A more complete discussion of infection in pregnancy will be presented in Chap. 14.

Vaccines Recommended in All Pregnancies

Influenza

Influenza is one of the illnesses that poses a significant risk to pregnant women. Unfortunately, the influenza vaccine also has likely the greatest amount of entrenched belief which can make it more difficult to counsel patients. Providers should ask each individual patient their concerns so that these can be addressed and an informed decision made. Pregnant women are at a significantly increased risk of severe complications from influenza, so it is of significant importance to counsel all pregnant patients on the benefits of receiving appropriate vaccination during pregnancy. Influenza vaccine comes in two main types: inactivated influenza vaccine (IIV) and live attenuated influenza vaccine (LAIV). IIV is recommended for all pregnant women who are or will be pregnant during the influenza season. The use of LAIV is contraindicated during pregnancy due to the possibility of viral activation and acute illness.

Tetanus, Diphtheria, and Pertussis (Tdap)

Tdap vaccine during pregnancy is of dual benefit. It will help ensure protection for the mother from a respiratory illness that can cause significant morbidity, and it provides postpartum protection for the infant until they can receive their first set of vaccines. Current recommendations are that pregnant patients receive the Tdap vaccine between 27 and 37 weeks of gestation for optimal antibody transfer to the newborn. Beyond 37 weeks giving the Tdap vaccine still provides maternal protection, though with the loss of antibody protection for the newborn. It is also important to recognize, for both the Tdap and IIV, that vaccination of close relatives can help to greatly decrease the newborn's risk of exposure, so should be encouraged.

Vaccines to Be Considered Based on Risk vs. Benefit

Hepatitis A

Hepatitis A can cause significant morbidity though most patients in developed nations are at low risk of exposure. However, if local rates of hepatitis A or patient exposure risks are unacceptably high, one would consider vaccinating. The safety of hepatitis A vaccination during pregnancy has yet to be determined, but as it is inactivated, the theoretic risk to the mother and fetus is thought to be low. If your pregnant patient is considering travelling to an area with increased prevalence of hepatitis A, a discussion regarding the possible need for this vaccine would be prudent.

Yellow Fever

Yellow fever is a severe illness present in subtropical Africa and South America. Though it is a live vaccine, it may be considered in pregnant women who have unavoidable travel to an endemic area. A clear discussion of maternal and fetal risks and benefits would be paramount prior to vaccine administration.

Meningococcal (B)

Meningococcal B strain meningitis is a severe, potentially life-threatening, illness with peak incidence in the young adult years, 16–23 years of age. Vaccination with MenB should be deferred unless the patient is at significant risk and would be considered only after a discussion between the provider and patient regarding risks and benefits.

Vaccines for Use if Indicated

For the following vaccines, there are recommendations that exposed patients receive them. For up-to-date recommendations and guidelines, please refer to current CDC/ACIP guidelines. Meningococcal (ACWY), polio, Td, anthrax, rabies, and smallpox

Vaccines Contraindicated in Pregnancy

Both the MMR and varicella vaccines are live attenuated vaccines. Similar to the LAIV, the risks to the fetus are too great, and pregnant women, or women expecting to become pregnant in the next month, should not be vaccinated with these vaccines. Finally, zoster vaccines should be avoided in pregnancy because firstly its risks are unknown and secondly this vaccine isn't recommended until 50 years of age.

Part II
Complications in Pregnancy

Chapter 6
Dysmorphic Growth and Genetic Abnormalities

Contents

Background... 47
History.. 48
Physical Examination.. 49
Diagnosis... 49
Obstetrical Screening Tests.. 50
    What Is Measured... 50
    What Is Detected... 50
    Confirmation/Follow-Up... 51
    Amniocentesis.. 51
    Chorionic Villus Sampling.. 52

> **Key Points**
> 1. Growth and development represent a complex interaction between genetic predisposition and environmental exposure.
> 2. Screening for genetic risk factors ideally begins in the preconception period.
> 3. Prenatal genetic testing is more nuanced than ever, and counseling should be approached in an organized fashion.

Background

Most fetuses are free from identifiable genetic abnormalities. Their pattern of growth and development falls within the range of normal parameters. Under some circumstances, physical growth is restricted (intrauterine growth restriction). This is discussed in Chap. 8. Under other circumstances, however, genetic abnormalities lead to abnormalities in growth, development, or both. These abnormalities may be relatively minor (e.g., color blindness) or they might be more significant (e.g., muscular dystrophy). Primary care providers must be familiar with common abnormalities and available screening options to identify these conditions when they arise. Routine fetal assessment has expanded greatly since its inception and especially notably in the past 10 years. Patients are often unaware of options available to them and the implications that these tests can have for the pregnancy and beyond. It is vitally important to be aware of and counsel on all recommended methods for prenatal assessment as an oversight could lead to a potentially missed diagnosis of congenital disorders. Providers need to be aware of all available screening methods in order to fully and correctly counsel their patients of their options for genetic screening.

Genetic inheritance is a complex interaction of maternal and paternal genotypic predisposition with a variety of environmental factors. The resulting phenotypic expression represents the final outcome of these two factors. A review of both familial genetic predisposition and environmental risk factors will allow providers to discuss with expectant parents the developmental risks, if any, associated with a particular pregnancy.

Chromosomal abnormalities fall within two major groups, abnormalities of chromosomal number (e.g., trisomy 21, Down syndrome) and abnormalities of chromosomal structure (e.g., hemophilia). Chromosomal abnormalities (genotypes) may have variable phenotypes. This variability can represent variable expressivity (variation in expression of a disease within a population with a specified genetic abnormality) and/or variable penetrance (likelihood of expression within an individual with a genetic abnormality).

History

Ideally genetic screening by history would begin in the preconception period. If that is not possible, it should begin as early in the prenatal period as possible. A variety of standardized screening tools exist to assist providers with the evaluation of maternal and paternal genetic risk factors. Table 6.1 provides a selected list of conditions commonly screened for in pregnancy. Common medical conditions with a strong genetic predisposition should be reviewed, including congenital abnormalities, cystic fibrosis, Down syndrome, hemophilia, sickle cell disease, neural tube defects, Tay–Sachs disease, and muscular dystrophy, among others. Although these standardized screening tools are helpful as a starting point, providers should be aware that additional detail may be required for some high-risk patients. If the primary care provider does not feel adequately prepared to complete such a genetic screening, referral should be made to a genetics counselor or a maternal–fetal medicine specialist.

In addition to a thorough family history, a history of recurrent early spontaneous abortions should be noted if present. Approximately 50% of early spontaneous

Table 6.1 Selected congenital conditions screened for in preconception/prenatal care	Endocrine disease
	Autoimmune disease
	Congenital abnormalities
	Cleft lip/palate
	Congenital heart disease
	Cystic fibrosis
	Down syndrome
	Mental retardation
	Neural tube defects
	Hemophilia
	Sickle cell disease
	Thalassemia
	Huntington's chorea
	Tay–Sachs disease

abortions are estimated to demonstrate genetic abnormalities. The age of the mother should be noted, as fetal genetic abnormalities increase with increasing maternal age. The prevalence of such disorders ranges from approximately 2 per 1000 live births at a maternal age of 25 years to approximately 150 per 1000 by maternal age 50.

Physical Examination

Although a physical examination may, rarely, uncover a genetic abnormality not discovered through careful history taking, in general the physical examination contributes little to the assessment of risk for genetic abnormalities.

Diagnosis

Although careful historical screening will identify many patients at risk for genetic and/or developmental abnormalities, adjunctive diagnostic testing is available and should be offered during the course of prenatal care. A wide variety of screening options are available, and patients requiring specialized testing should be managed in conjunction with a genetics counselor and an experienced maternal–fetal medicine specialist. Three such tests (obstetrical triple screen, amniocentesis, chorionic villus sampling [CVS]), however, are offered with sufficient frequency that all primary care providers should be familiar with their basic function.

Obstetrical Screening Tests

First trimester combined test, first and second trimester combined test, and cell-free DNA

What Is Measured

This test measures maternal serum levels of pregnancy-associated plasma protein A, human chorionic gonadotropin, in conjunction with an ultrasound measure of nuchal translucency (done between 10 and 14 weeks). Standardized values are established for these three components during weeks 10–14 and 15–18 of pregnancy. Screen positive results are followed by CVS or amniocentesis based on gestational age (see below).

In cell-free DNA, a maternal blood sample is taken at any gestational age after 10 weeks. This test is most sensitive for detecting Down syndrome but can detect other major aneuploidies. At this time, it is recommended for use in women at higher risk for trisomy 21. While it does have higher accuracy when used in the correct population, cell-free DNA is still a screening test, and confirmatory CVS or amniocentesis is still needed.

What Is Detected

Down Syndrome

Down syndrome is a genetic abnormality of abnormal chromosomal distribution (trisomy) associated developmentally with mental retardation of variable degree, characteristic physical stigmata, and an association with a variety of other medical conditions including cardiac and hematological diseases. The prevalence of Down syndrome increases with increasing maternal age and with prior history of Down syndrome.

Down syndrome should be suspected with abnormally low triple screen results. Triple screen testing will identify approximately 60% of all cases of Down syndrome. Although this is sufficiently sensitive for low-risk populations, higher-risk populations may require more accurate testing methods (see the next section). Abnormally, low triple screen testing is falsely positive in approximately 5% of cases. The most common cause of false-positive testing is inaccurate gestational dating.

Neural Tube Defects

Although the serum tests of this screen can be correlated with the risk of neural tube defect, it is more accurately measured during the second trimester.

Confirmation/Follow-Up

Triple screen testing is, by definition, a screening test, and all abnormal values require confirmation and diagnostic follow-up. For all abnormal values, confirmation of gestational age is critical. All data used to establish the gestational age should be reviewed and confirmed. Under some circumstances, repeat triple screening may be indicated.

Confirmed abnormal elevations in triple screen results should be followed up with obstetrical ultrasound. This study will allow for careful examination of the anatomy of the developing fetus. In addition, ultrasonographic studies should allow for identification of multigestation and fetal demise.

Confirmed abnormally low triple screen results should be followed by genetics counseling with amniocentesis and fetal karyotyping.

Amniocentesis

Amniocentesis is a diagnostic procedure that consists of introduction of a sampling needle through the abdominal wall into the amniotic sac. A small sample of amniotic fluid is withdrawn, allowing for a variety of potential studies. The most common study performed with the fluid is determination of the fetal karyotype.

As noted earlier, an abnormal low triple screen is one indication for amniocentesis. Other indications include maternal age over 35 years, prior chromosomal abnormality, three or more prior spontaneous abortions, and known parental chromosomal abnormality.

Amniocentesis can be performed between 12 and 17 weeks' gestation. The risk of complications is higher earlier in pregnancy. For this reason, most are performed between 15 and 17 weeks' gestation. The most significant complication associated with amniocentesis is spontaneous abortion. The reported rate of post-amniocentesis spontaneous abortion is approximately 1 per 200 procedures, although the risk may be significantly lower in settings with highly experienced operators. Sensitivity and specificity are both >99%.

Chorionic Villus Sampling

The need to wait until 15 weeks' gestation represents a significant limitation for amniocentesis in some cases. For this reason, alternative methods that may be performed earlier have been developed. One such method is CVS. The procedure is performed via transcervical or transabdominal approach with the target being at least 5 mg of chorionic villus tissue. CVS may be performed in earlier than amniocentesis (after 10 weeks' gestation) with similar sensitivity, specificity, and complication rates. Indications for CVS include:

1. Maternal age > 35
2. Prior chromosomal abnormality
3. Positive serum screening test
4. Ultrasonographic abnormality
5. Parental chromosomal abnormality

Chapter 7
Intrauterine Growth Restriction

Contents

Background.. 53
Risk Factors... 55
  Fetal–Genetic Factors... 55
  Uterine–Environmental Factors... 55
  Maternal Factors... 56
  Toxic Exposures.. 56
  Constitutional Factors.. 57
Complications of Growth Restriction... 57
Antenatal Tracking and Diagnosis.. 57
Screening for Risks.. 59
Diagnosis.. 60
Management.. 60
  Risk Reduction.. 60

Key Points

1. Intrauterine growth restriction (IUGR) is defined as fetal weight below the 10th percentile and an abdominal girth below the 2.5 percentile.
2. Factors associated with IUGR can be categorized as fetal–genetic, uterine–environmental, maternal, toxic exposures, and constitutional.
3. Complications associated with IUGR include early complications (increased mortality, pre-eclampsia, preterm labor, still birth) and late complications (learning, behavioral, and developmental abnormalities).

Background

Fetal growth is among the most important of parameters monitored during the course of prenatal care. Although the majority of pregnancies proceed with no complications in fetal growth, a small number will show evidence of growth restriction.

© Springer Nature Switzerland AG 2020
P. Lyons, N. McLaughlin, *Obstetrics in Family Medicine*, Current Clinical Practice,
https://doi.org/10.1007/978-3-030-39888-0_7

Table 7.1 Risk factors for intrauterine growth restriction (IUGR)

Fetal–genetic factors
Chromosomal abnormalities (e.g., trisomy 21)
Neural tube defects
Achondroplasia
Osteogenesis imperfecta
Gastrointestinal (gastroschisis, duodenal atresia, pancreatic agenesis)
Renal disease (renal agenesis)
Neurofibromatosis
Uterine–environmental factors
Infection
Cytomegalovirus
Rubella
Herpes, varicella
Influenza
Toxoplasmosis
Oligohydramnios
Placental abnormalities
Placenta previa
Abruptio placentae
Placental malformation
Multigestation
Uterine anatomic abnormalities
Maternal factors
Prior IUGR infant
Hypertension
Diabetes (may also be associated with macrosomic infants)
Nutritional deficits
Gastrointestinal malabsorption
Constitutional short stature
Vascular disease
Toxic exposures
Smoking
Alcohol
Illicit drugs (heroin, cocaine)
Prescription medications (folic acid antagonists, warfarin)
Constitutional
Constitutional short stature
Female
Birth order

A variety of conditions are associated with or increase the risk for intrauterine growth restriction (IUGR). These factors are summarized in Table 7.1.

IUGR and small for gestational age (SGA) although often overlapping are defined somewhat differently. IUGR is defined clinically by evidence of growth rate restriction (symmetric or asymmetric) with evidence of growth retardation and/or malnutrition. Under some circumstances, there may be evidence of growth restriction in infants with average for gestational age (AGA) weight. Small for gestational age (SGA) is defined as any infant below the 10th percentile for gestational age as fetal weight below the 10th percentile with or without clinical evidence of malnutrition or growth restriction other than weight. Despite this distinction, for practical purposes, IUGR is often defined as <10th percentile weight and an abdominal girth below the 2.5th percentile for gestational age. As this definition implies, accurate fetal dating is critical to the diagnosis. At term, this corresponds to a birth weight of 2500 g (~5.5 lb). By this definition, approximately 5% of all US infants demonstrate evidence of IUGR, accounting for approximately 175,000 infants annually in the United States.

Fetal growth assessment generally includes measurement of biparietal diameter, femur length, and abdominal girth. IUGR can be classified as either symmetric (restriction of approximately equal degree in all growth parameters) or asymmetric (restriction of unequal degree among growth parameters). Symmetric IUGR comprises approximately 25% of all cases, generally reflects an insult earlier in pregnancy, and is often indicative of genetic or infectious etiology. Asymmetric IUGR is more common (~75% of all cases), generally reflects a later onset, and is most commonly associated with utero-placental insufficiency. Although there is high variability postpartum, the prognosis is less good for symmetric IUGR.

Risk Factors

Factors associated with IUGR can be categorized into five categories: fetal–genetic, uterine–environmental, maternal, toxic exposures, and constitutional factors.

Fetal–Genetic Factors

A variety of genetic conditions are associated with restricted fetal growth and account for approximately 10% of all cases. Early fetal growth is predominantly driven by growth in the number of fetal cells, cellular hyperplasia. This process is strongly influenced by genetic and fetal factors. As such early growth restriction is predominantly associated with fetal–genetic factors. Such conditions as Down syndrome (trisomy 21) and Turner's syndrome are associated with an increased risk for IUGR. Structural growth defects such as anencephaly, achondroplasia, osteogenesis imperfecta, and renal and gastrointestinal (GI) defects are all associated with an increased risk of IUGR.

Uterine–Environmental Factors

Abnormalities of the uterine environment may also contribute to growth restriction. Congenital infections such as cytomegalovirus, toxoplasmosis, or rubella are associated with restricted fetal growth. Although these infections can cause significant fetal growth restriction, they are a relatively uncommon cause of IUGR, <5%. Fetal urinary tract outflow obstruction with concomitant oligohydramnios can be associated with IUGR. Placental abnormalities (placenta previa, abruption, placental malformation) and multiple gestations can both alter the uterine environment and therefore lead to growth restriction. The structure of the uterus itself may also contribute to growth restriction. Utero-placental insufficiency is most commonly associated with late-onset growth restriction.

Maternal Factors

Growth in pregnancy is fundamentally reliant on a balance between fetal needs (especially nutrition and oxygen) and maternal ability to meet those needs. Following the period of cellular hyperplasia, fetal growth is augmented by cellular hypertrophy. Growth restriction due to decreased cellular hypertrophy may be more responsive to correction of nutritional imbalances. Maternal health and nutrition contribute significantly to fetal growth, and a number of maternal factors can be associated with decreased fetal growth. Although specific maternal factors may not always be identified, a pregnant patient with a past history of IUGR is approximately twice as likely to have subsequent IUGR compared to those without such a history. Prepregnancy maternal factors that may be identified include age (<16 or >35), weight (BMI <20), parity (nulliparous or >5 prior births), and short interpregnancy interval (<6 months).

Underlying maternal diseases such as diabetes, hypertension, GI, and vascular disease are all associated with an increased risk for IUGR. Hypertension is associated with decreased placental perfusion resulting in decreased delivery of both oxygen and nutrients. GI disease with significant malabsorption will result in decreased delivery of nutrients to the fetus and may contribute to subsequent IUGR. It should be noted that less significant nutritional defects may not result in diminished fetal growth as nutrients are delivered preferentially to the fetus.

Fetal growth is dependent on adequate fetal oxygenation and delivery of necessary nutrients. Adequate delivery is dependent, in turn, on adequate vascular function. Maternal vascular disease associated with a number of diseases impairs maternal–fetal perfusion and therefore is associated with increased risk of IUGR. Such maternal conditions as diabetes mellitus, peripheral vascular disease associated with tobacco use, collagen vascular disease, and pregnancy complications such as pre-eclampsia can all decrease maternal–fetal perfusion, thus increasing the risk of IUGR.

Toxic Exposures

The use of toxic substances (tobacco, alcohol, and illicit drugs) has been associated with decreased fetal growth. Of these, tobacco use is by far the most common risk factor for diminished fetal growth. Pregnant patients who smoke approximately double the risk of IUGR, a risk that is proportional to the quantity of cigarettes smoked. Discontinuation of smoking before or during pregnancy is associated with reduction or elimination of this risk. Both alcohol and illicit drug use (especially heroin and cocaine) are associated with diminished fetal growth. Fetal alcohol syndrome infants are generally small for gestational age.

Prescription drug use may also be associated with decreased fetal growth. Folic acid is a critical component in fetal development. Supplementation with folate is recommended during the preconception and early prenatal course. Drugs that inhibit folic acid metabolism may result in decreased fetal growth among other complications. The use of warfarin for anticoagulation has also been associated with IUGR.

Constitutional Factors

Small mothers are more likely to have small infants. Although these infants are small for gestational age, they are otherwise healthy. If no maternal, fetal, or uterine factors can be identified, these infants are generally healthy and normal but small. It is estimated that 50% or more of SGA infants are of appropriate size for gender, ethnicity, and maternal size. There is some variation in size based on birth order and gender. First infants are slightly smaller, on average, than subsequent infants; female infants are somewhat smaller, on average, than male infants.

Complications of Growth Restriction

Although not all small babies have complications, IUGR represents the second leading cause of perinatal morbidity and mortality after prematurity. Infants with a birth weight below 2500 g have a mortality rate of 5–30 times that of infants weighing more than 2500 g. IUGR (or associated underlying disease processes) is associated with an increased risk for pre-eclampsia, preterm labor/delivery, stillbirth, fetal electrolyte abnormalities, hypoglycemia, hypothermia, polycythemia, and aspiration. Long-term consequences associated with IUGR include increased risk for learning, behavioral, and developmental abnormalities.

Antenatal Tracking and Diagnosis

Every prenatal visit includes assessment of fetal growth either indirectly or directly. A general approach to tracking fetal growth is presented in Fig. 7.1. Indirect measures of fetal growth include maternal weight gain, fundal height, and age-appropriate landmarks (e.g., fetal heart tones heard with handheld Doppler at approximately 10–12 weeks' gestation). Direct measures of fetal growth can be obtained with obstetrical ultrasound. Interpretation of these markers depends on

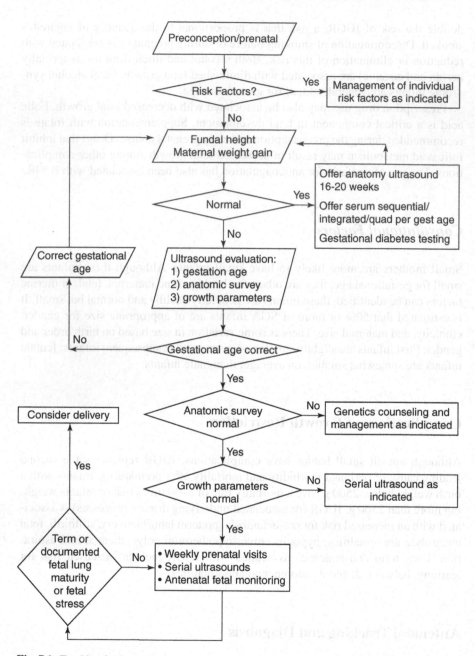

Fig. 7.1 Tracking fetal growth

accurate pregnancy dating. Parameters for establishing gestational age and estimated date of delivery (EDD) are covered in Chap. 3. In addition to assessing markers of fetal growth, all patients should be screened for risk factors that may contribute to an increased risk for IUGR.

Screening for Risks

The first prenatal visit will include a comprehensive historical review of the patient's, patient's family, and paternal risk factors. Particular note should be made of prior obstetrical history, including infant size at delivery, prior history of genetic abnormalities including neural tube defects and Down syndrome, and multiple gestations. The mother's history should be reviewed for chronic disease such as hypertension, cardiovascular disease, renal disease, diabetes mellitus (including prior macrosomic infants with or without a known diagnosis of diabetes mellitus), GI disease, and nutritional status. The note should be made of alcohol, tobacco, or illicit drug use.

Physical examination at the first prenatal visit should include assessment of uterine size (and comparison of this finding to estimated gestational age). If appropriate, fetal heart tones should be documented at this visit. Initial laboratory studies that may contribute to risk screening would include protein or glucose on urinalysis and evidence of cytomegalovirus, herpes, rubella, and/or toxoplasmosis.

Each subsequent visit will include interval updates for each of these risk factors. Patients should be screened for changes in nutritional status, toxic substance use, medications, or new exposures. Each prenatal visit will include documentation of blood pressure, maternal weight, fundal height, and fetal heart rate. Particular attention should be paid to fundal height measurement as this can be a significant clue to growth abnormalities. Fundal height (measured symphysis pubis to top of fundus) in centimeters should be equal to gestational age in weeks (±2 cm).

At 15–20 weeks' gestation, patients should be offered α-fetoprotein (or triple test) screening. Also, in this time period, many patients will undergo obstetrical ultrasound examination. Key parameters on ultrasound include biparietal diameter, head circumference, abdominal girth, estimated fetal weight, and amniotic fluid index (AFI). Routine screening for gestational diabetes is performed at 24–28 weeks' gestation but may be performed earlier in patients with increased risk.

Patients who show abnormalities in any of these parameters should be considered at increased risk for IUGR with appropriate follow-up and diagnostic testing when indicated.

Diagnosis

Diagnosis of IUGR requires correlation of gestational age with ultrasonographic measurements of fetal growth. The accuracy of the diagnosis is ultimately dependent on the accuracy of each of these components. IUGR must also be understood to be a *growth* phenomenon; a single static measurement may be suggestive but is not diagnostic. Serial measurements are generally required to diagnose IUGR.

Estimation of gestational age is based on the last menstrual period, key developmental markers (such as heartbeat), and sonographic data. Sonographic data can be useful for three purposes: (a) estimation of gestational age, (b) identification of structural or developmental abnormalities, and (c) measurement of fetal growth parameters. The most accurate ultrasound parameters for estimating gestational age vary with the age of the fetus. Crown–rump length is most accurate in early pregnancy; biparietal diameter and head circumference are most accurate for second trimester evaluation. Third trimester estimates are decreasingly accurate, but head circumference may be most accurate. The increased sophistication of obstetrical ultrasounds has yielded images capable of remarkable anatomic detail. Cardiac, renal, GI, and neurological anomalies may all be detected on ultrasound examination. Patients with suspected IUGR should undergo ultrasound examination with particular attention paid to detailed anatomic survey.

In addition to the parameters mentioned here, abdominal girth is particularly helpful in measuring fetal growth. Abdominal girth reflects subcutaneous fat that, in turn, is a marker for adequate fetal nutrition. IUGR is often associated with an oligohydramnios (decreased amniotic fluid) that can be measured via the AFI. The AFI is the sum of the largest fluid pocket in each of the four quadrants. IUGR with oligohydramnios is associated with increased morbidity compared with IUGR alone.

Although not diagnostic of IUGR, measurement of fetal vascular flow, Doppler velocimetry, can provide additional clinical information regarding fetal well-being. Blood flow is measured in the umbilical artery, and the ratio of systolic to diastolic flow is calculated. Peak systolic frequency shift/end-diastolic frequency shift (*S/D*) ratios of 1.8–2.0 are normal. *S/D* ratios >3.0 indicate a pregnancy at high risk for adverse outcomes. Measurement of flow can also be measured in the middle cerebral artery and the ductus venosus.

Management

Risk Reduction

Although early identification and management can reduce the morbidity associated with IUGR, risk reduction remains a critical component of management. Ideally, such risk evaluation and reduction would begin in the preconception period with identification of pre-existing risk factors. For patients with a strong history of genetic abnormalities, genetics counseling may be indicated prior to conception. Identification of pre-existing medical conditions and nutritional deficits may also contribute to a reduction in the risk for IUGR. Although the benefits of such management in IUGR have not been well established, control of blood pressure, euglycemia prior to conception, and nutritional augmentation, among others, are recommended. Patients who smoke should be counseled to discontinue smoking; alcohol use should also be discontinued. The use of illicit drugs should be identified, and cessation should be counseled. For many patients, pregnancy may represent a compelling reason to reduce or discontinue the use of toxic substances with benefit to both the mother and fetus.

Infectious risks for IUGR should be reviewed with the patient and reduction of exposure counseled. Toxoplasmosis is associated with raw or undercooked meat and cat feces. Patients should be counseled concerning exposure to those with varicella and rubella. If patients are seen in the preconceptual period, immune status should be documented for varicella and rubella. Vaccinations for both are available and should be administered to nonimmune patients who do not plan to become pregnant in the subsequent 3 months.

With diagnosis of IUGR, management involves three basic tasks: (a) identification and modification (when possible) of underlying etiology, (b) monitoring for anticipated or possible complications, and (c) evaluation of risks and benefits of continued pregnancy versus early delivery. Identification of the potential etiology is similar to preconception evaluation. The benefits of intervention are not well documented, but management of medical conditions such as hypertension and diabetes, augmentation of nutritional status, and reduction or elimination of tobacco, alcohol, and illicit drug use are recommended.

Complications associated with IUGR include prenatal and perinatal complications such as increased risk of hypoxia, metabolic acidosis, preterm labor, preeclampsia, and surgical delivery. Neonatal complications include aspiration, apnea, intubation, sepsis, hypoglycemia, electrolyte abnormalities (especially hypocalcemia), seizure, and death. Careful intrapartum monitoring is critical to early identification and management of these potential complications.

In patients with documented IUGR, careful assessment of fetal growth and well-being is critical to determining the timing and manner of delivery. Weekly prenatal visits are recommended, with careful monitoring of fetal status with review of fetal movement and kick counts. As noted, serial measurements (every 2–6 weeks) of fetal growth are important for the diagnosis as well as for tracking. Antenatal fetal monitoring may also include nonstress testing, contraction stress testing, and/or biophysical profile measurements at least weekly. Amniotic fluid should be measured via AFI once weekly.

Management of IUGR requires individualized assessment and decision-making. Timing of delivery should balance the benefits of further fetal maturity against the risks of continued exposure to an intrauterine environment that is less than optimal. Evidence of fetal maturity (well-documented gestational age of 38 weeks' gestation or documentation of fetal lung maturity) or significant fetal stress should prompt delivery. For infants with reassuring antenatal monitoring and without evidence of maturity, the benefits of intrauterine development may outweigh the risks of early delivery. Delivery should be planned for a facility that is experienced with and capable of managing the high-risk infants of a pregnancy complicated by IUGR. Management of perinatal complications in the infant is best managed by an experienced neonatologist.

Chapter 8
Preterm Labor

Contents

Background... 64
Factors Associated with Preterm Labor.................................... 64
Preconception Factor... 65
   Environmental Factors.. 65
   Patient-Related Factors... 65
Postconception Factors.. 65
Diagnosis.. 66
Intake Assessment.. 66
   History.. 66
   Physical Examination... 67
   Laboratory Studies.. 67
Management... 67
   Management Prior to 34 Weeks' Gestation........................... 69
   Management at 34–37 Weeks... 70
Assessment of Fetal Lung Maturity... 70
   Lecithin-to-Sphingomyelin Ratio...................................... 71
   Phosphatidylglycerol.. 71
   Additional Tests... 71

> **Key Points**
> 1. Preterm labor is uterine contractions resulting in progressive cervical change prior to 37 weeks' gestation. Preterm delivery is delivery prior to 37 weeks' gestation; low-birth weight infants are those that weigh less than 2500 g at delivery.
> 2. Prior to 34 weeks' gestation, most patients should be considered for tocolysis; from 34 to 37 weeks' gestation, such decisions must be made on a case-by-case basis.
> 3. Complications associated with preterm delivery include increased perinatal mortality and complications of prematurity (including respiratory distress, gastrointestinal dysfunction, hemorrhage, and abnormalities of growth and development).

© Springer Nature Switzerland AG 2020
P. Lyons, N. McLaughlin, *Obstetrics in Family Medicine*, Current Clinical Practice,
https://doi.org/10.1007/978-3-030-39888-0_8

Background

Preterm labor is among the most common and most serious of prenatal complications. Preterm labor and its potential sequelae of preterm delivery and low-birth weight (LBW) infants remain one of the most significant challenges of current obstetrical practice. Preterm labor is defined as uterine contractions resulting in progressive cervical change prior to 37 weeks' gestation. Preterm delivery is delivery prior to 37 weeks' gestation. LBW infants are defined as those infants weighing less than 2500 g at delivery regardless of gestational age. LBW infants should be distinguished from small-for-gestational-age (SGA) infants who are defined as those infants below the tenth percentile for weight based on gestational age.

Preterm labor affects approximately 10% of all pregnancies. Preterm delivery affects approximately 13% of all live births. Preterm delivery and LBW infants represent approximately 70% of all perinatal mortality (~25,000 deaths annually) and 50% of all neurological morbidity.

Factors Associated with Preterm Labor

A number of factors have been associated with an increased risk of preterm labor. These are summarized in Table 8.1. These factors can be divided into pre- and post-conception factors. Although the mechanisms that link these factors to the onset of preterm labor are, in most instances, poorly understood, a thorough review of the patient's history will allow providers to more carefully outline the risk of preterm labor, preterm delivery, and LBW infants.

Table 8.1 Risk factors for preterm labor

Preconception factors
Lower socioeconomic status
Anatomic abnormalities (e.g., septate/bicornuate uterus, cervical incompetence)
Prior uterine surgery
Myomata
Diethylstilbestrol exposure
Past history of preterm labor
Under 18 years old, over 40 years old
Possible genetic predisposition
Postconception factors
Tobacco
Cocaine
Infection (e.g., group B streptococcus, *N. gonorrhoeae*, *C. trachomatis*, trichomonas, gardnerella, ureaplasma, mycoplasma)

Although preterm labor alone is not associated with perinatal complications, concomitant conditions and outcomes are. Preterm labor may be complicated by preterm premature rupture of membranes (PPROM). PPROM is associated with a variety of complications discussed in Chap. 8. Preterm labor may also result in preterm delivery. Prematurity, in turn, is potentially associated with pulmonary dysfunction, gastrointestinal abnormalities, neurological complications, abnormalities of growth and development, and a significant risk of perinatal mortality. Complications of preterm delivery are the leading cause of perinatal mortality, responsible for approximately two-thirds of all deaths.

Preconception Factor

Environmental Factors

A number of environmental factors have been associated with an increased risk of preterm labor. The most significant environmental factor associated with preterm labor is lower socioeconomic status.

Patient-Related Factors

A number of pre-existing patient conditions also contribute to the risk of preterm labor. Patients may have a pre-existing genetic risk, a congenital anomaly (e.g., septate/bicornuate uterus, or cervical incompetence), a pre-existing acquired obstetrical/gynecological risk (e.g., myomata, uterine surgery, diethylstilbestrol exposure), or a past history of preterm labor or second trimester spontaneous abortions. The recurrence rate of preterm labor is approximately 25%. Additionally, the risk of preterm labor is highest among younger (<18 years old) and older (>40 years old) obstetrical patients. These conditions can be screened for early in pregnancy (or during preconception counseling). Although many of these factors are not modifiable, their presence can usefully contribute to a conversation between the provider and the patient concerning the risk for preterm labor during the current pregnancy.

Postconception Factors

Once conception occurs, a number of additional factors contribute to the risk of preterm labor. An increased risk for preterm labor is associated with tobacco and cocaine use. Infections such as group B streptococcus, gonorrhea, chlamydia, trichomonas, gardnerella, ureaplasma, and mycoplasma have all been associated with increased preterm labor risk. Such exposures should be screened for at the first prenatal history (either directly through testing or via history) and as appropriate throughout the course of pregnancy.

Diagnosis

As noted earlier, the diagnosis of preterm labor consists of three components: gestational age less than 37 weeks, presence of uterine contractions, and progressive cervical change.

The diagnosis of preterm labor begins with confirmation of the gestational age of the fetus. All data that contributed to the estimated date of delivery (EDD) should be reviewed for accuracy. The patient's last menstrual period should be reviewed for accuracy. Additional data such as prenatal ultrasound, sequential fundal height measurements, and gestational age at quickening should also be reviewed. If no such data is available, an obstetrical ultrasound may be indicated. It should be emphasized, however, that an ultrasound obtained late in pregnancy has significantly less accuracy for purposes of gestational dating.

The patient should be questioned concerning the presence of contractions (although the absence of patient-reported contractions does not exclude the possibility of clinically significant contractile activity). If preterm labor is suspected, patients should be placed on tocometric monitoring to confirm the presence of uterine contractions.

Documentation of progressive cervical change, under most circumstances, requires serial cervical examinations. After confirming the absence of bleeding per vagina, providers should document cervical dilation and effacement as well as fetal station. Although the patient may demonstrate unequivocal cervical evidence of labor on initial examination, generally, the diagnosis will require comparison of initial findings to findings on a follow-up examination.

Intake Assessment

History

In addition to the history noted earlier, patients should be asked about bleeding per vagina, rupture of membranes or fluid leak, and/or symptoms of infection. Special caution should be exercised if the patient reports a history of bleeding per vagina. The management of third-trimester bleeding is covered in Chap. 10. A review of the past history should note the presence of cardiac, renal pulmonary, and/or endocrine abnormalities.

Physical Examination

In addition to the pelvic examination for assessment of cervical change, the intake physical examination should document blood pressure, pulse, temperature, rupture of membranes (see Chap. 8), fetal heart rate, and uterine contractions.

Laboratory Studies

Patients admitted with preterm labor should have all prenatal laboratory values reviewed with lab values ordered or updated as necessary. Patients may require testing for infection, including gonorrhea, chlamydia, group B strep trichomonas, and bacterial vaginosis. Other studies that may contribute to evaluation of possible infection include increased interleukin-6 in amniotic or cervical samples, elevated ferritin in cervical or serum samples, and elevated granulocyte colony-stimulating factor in serum samples. Patients demonstrating clinical signs or symptoms of other obstetrical conditions (e.g., pregnancy-induced hypertension) should have laboratory evaluation as indicated for those conditions.

Controversy exists concerning the role of routine fibronectin testing in the management of suspected preterm labor. Specimens should be obtained via sterile speculum examination. A swab is placed in the posterior fornix for 10 s. Care should be taken to avoid manipulation of the cervix or use of lubricant. Known rupture of membranes is a contraindication to fibronectin testing. After 22 weeks' gestation, a result greater than 50 ng/mL is associated with an increased risk for preterm delivery with a sensitivity of 70–90% and a specificity of 70–85%. The negative predictive value is approximately 99%. A negative test is a strong predictor of no preterm labor in the week following the test. Fetal breathing movements and measurement of cervical length can be used in conjunction with or as an alternative to fibronectin testing. Fibronectin has been shown to have the highest sensitivity and fetal breathing movement the highest specificity for delivery within 7 days of testing. In patients with a cervical length >30 mm, risk of delivery within 7 days is less than 5%, and fibronectin does not add to diagnostic accuracy.

Management

The management of preterm labor is often limited in efficacy and duration, and few modifiable factors have been identified. A general outline of management is shown in Fig. 8.1. Goals of management are focused on delay of delivery to allow four key outcomes:

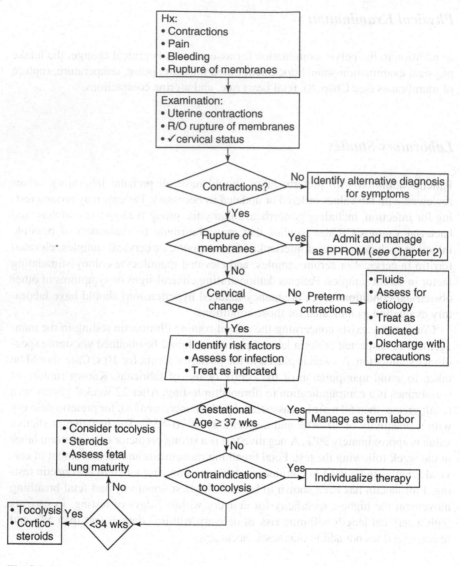

Fig. 8.1 Management of preterm labor

1. Transfer, if necessary, to a facility with appropriate neonatal intensive care services
2. Administration of corticosteroids to decrease postpartum complications for the infant
3. Administration of magnesium sulfate (associated with a decreased risk of cerebral palsy)
4. Administration of appropriate prophylaxis for group B strep

Decisions concerning appropriate management should be tailored to the individual patient. Despite the challenge and variability involved in managing preterm labor, a few general guidelines can be given.

Management Prior to 34 Weeks' Gestation

In general, fetal lung maturity cannot be assumed in infants prior to 34 weeks' gestation. For this reason, tocolysis is generally recommended. Although the efficacy and duration of such therapy are limited, a brief delay in delivery allows for administration of corticosteroids to enhance fetal lung maturity. All patients should be screened for contraindications to tocolysis (see Table 8.2). Contraindications to tocolysis include underlying medical contraindications (cardiac disease, renal insufficiency, pyelonephritis, pulmonary hypertension, untreated diabetes mellitus, and electrolyte abnormalities) and obstetrical contraindications (fetal stress, chorioamnionitis, eclampsia, fetal demise, and hemodynamic instability). Tocolytic options include the following:

1. Terbutaline (β-2-sympathomimetic): 250 μg subcutaneously every 3–4 h.
2. Ritodrine (β-2-sympathomimetic): 100 μg per minute intravenous starting dose. Dose increased 50 μg per minute every 20 min until contractions cease.
3. Magnesium sulfate ($MgSO_4$): 6 g intravenous load over 15 min then 2 g per hour. It may be increased every hour until contractions cease, maximum dose of 5 g per hour is reached, or signs or symptoms of magnesium toxicity occur. Magnesium toxicity may be noted as neurological depression, cardiac depression or arrest, tetany, and hypotension. Monitoring of all patients on magnesium should include serum magnesium levels, maternal deep tendon reflexes, blood pressure, and strict recording of fluid input and output. Urinary retention is associated with magnesium use. Magnesium levels above 7 mEq/L are associated

Table 8.2 Contraindications to tocolysis	Medical contraindications
	Cardiac disease
	Renal insufficiency
	Pyelonephritis
	Pulmonary hypertension
	Untreated diabetes mellitus
	Electrolyte abnormalities
	Obstetrical contraindications
	Fetal stress
	Chorioamnionitis
	Eclampsia
	Fetal demise
	Hemodynamic instability

with diminished deep tendon reflexes, above 10 mEq/L with respiratory depression, and above 12 mEq/L with cardiac depression and arrest. Magnesium toxicity is treated with calcium gluconate 1 g intravenous.

4. Indomethacin (nonsteroidal anti-inflammatory, prostaglandin inhibitor): 100 mg per rectum or 50 mg orally loading dose and 50 mg per rectum or 25 mg orally every 4–6 h. Prior to 32 weeks, indomethacin has been shown to have equal efficacy to β-2-sympathomimetic agents probably by inhibiting prostaglandin synthesis. Use of indomethacin is associated with oligohydramnios and premature closure of the ductus arteriosus. For this reason, all patients on indomethacin should undergo frequent (every other day) ultrasound examinations to monitor for oligohydramnios. Because of the concern for premature ductus arteriosus closure, the use of indomethacin after 32 weeks gestation is controversial.

5. Nifedipine (calcium channel blockade): 20 mg orally loading dose and 10 mg orally every 6 h. Nifedipine's action in blocking calcium channel function in the smooth muscle is postulated to explain its efficacy in reducing uterine contractility. Studies have demonstrated efficacy similar to β-2-sympathomimetic agents.

Patients should be admitted and placed on bed rest. If significant cervical dilation has occurred, patients may be placed in a head-down position. Routine management includes monitoring of fluid status, hemodynamic status, and fetal well-being. If there is question concerning the gestational age or fetal lung status, fetal lung maturity testing may be considered. Mothers of infants at risk for fetal lung immaturity (24–35 weeks' gestation) should be treated with 12 mg of betamethasone, intramuscularly. Two doses should be given 24 h apart. Patients with evidence of contributory infection should be treated as appropriate for the infection.

Management at 34–37 Weeks

Fetal lung maturity in this range is highly variable, and decisions to initiate tocolysis must be individualized. When time permits, assessment of fetal lung maturity may assist in decisions concerning tocolysis versus expectant management.

Assessment of Fetal Lung Maturity

Delivery of an infant prior to fetal lung maturation is associated with considerable neonatal morbidity and mortality. For this reason, assessment of fetal lung maturity is critical in all instances where gestational age cannot be firmly established or when prenatal complications require consideration of an early delivery.

Confirmation of the gestational age is critical. Gestational age can be confirmed by review of the last menstrual period, early obstetrical ultrasound results, and key developmental milestones such as quickening and fetal heart tones. Although these data may allow for accurate gestational dating when available, not all data will be available in all cases. Even with such data, a more accurate assessment of fetal lung maturity may be necessary to guide management decisions. A variety of options are available to assist in this assessment.

Lecithin-to-Sphingomyelin Ratio

As fetal lung maturity progresses, pulmonary secretions are accumulated in the amniotic fluid allowing for assessment of fetal lung maturity based on amniotic fluid sampling. Lecithin and sphingomyelin are present in approximately equal quantities until approximately 8 weeks prior to the EDD. Beginning at this point, lecithin concentrations increase, and sphingomyelin concentrations remain stable. As the fetus nears maturation, therefore, the ratio of lecithin to sphingomyelin will increase. Although the exact interpretation of the results may be site dependent, a lecithin-to-sphingomyelin ratio of 2:1 or greater is associated with generally favorable neonatal pulmonary outcomes.

Phosphatidylglycerol

The presence of blood or meconium in the amniotic fluid may alter the results of the lecithin-to-sphingomyelin ratio. For this reason, alternative tests have been developed that are not sensitive to the presence of these substances. One such test is phosphatidylglycerol, a component of surfactant that is present in amniotic fluid and increases in quantity as fetal lung maturity advances. Amniotic fluid samples may be tested for phosphatidylglycerol alone or in conjunction with lecithin–sphingomyelin testing. The presence of phosphatidylglycerol is associated with more advanced fetal lung maturity and therefore with generally improved neonatal pulmonary outcomes. The results may be reported either qualitatively or quantitatively.

Additional Tests

Because of the importance of documenting fetal lung maturity and the complexity/limitations of traditionally available tests, a variety of alternative tests are now available. FLM-TDx II is a simple and reliable test (although it can be affected by blood or meconium). A value of >55 mg/g of albumin is considered indicative of fetal lung maturity. Lamellar body count (affected by blood but not meconium) with a value >50,000 is also indicative of fetal lung maturity.

Chapter 9
Premature Rupture of Membranes

Contents

Background.. 73
Diagnosis.. 74
   History... 74
   Physical Examination.. 75
   Laboratory.. 76
Management... 77
   Management at Term... 78
   Preterm Management.. 78

Key Points
1. Premature rupture of membranes (PROM) is defined as rupture prior to the onset of labor.
2. Preterm premature rupture of membranes (PPROM) is defined as PROM occurring prior to 37 weeks' gestation.
3. Rupture of membranes is followed by onset of labor within 24 h in 90% of term patients and 50% of preterm patients.
4. PROM is associated with an increased risk of ascending infection. This risk increases with duration of rupture.

Background

For most women, the pattern of labor is predictable. In general, women first note the onset of contractions that are relatively mild and irregular. As labor progresses, the contractions become stronger and more regular and of increased duration. Spontaneous rupture of membranes generally follows the development of a regular contraction pattern as cervical dilation progresses. In approximately 10% of cases, however, spontaneous rupture of membranes occurs prior to the onset of labor. This is defined as premature rupture of membranes (PROM).

© Springer Nature Switzerland AG 2020
P. Lyons, N. McLaughlin, *Obstetrics in Family Medicine*, Current Clinical Practice,
https://doi.org/10.1007/978-3-030-39888-0_9

Premature, in this case, does not refer to gestational age but to labor. If rupture of membranes precedes labor *and* is prior to 37 weeks' gestation, the condition is referred to as preterm premature rupture of membranes (PPROM). Rupture of membranes is generally followed by onset of labor within 24 h. Ninety percent of patients at term and 50% of preterm patients will begin labor within 24 h of spontaneous rupture of membranes. For term patients, PROM will generally mark impending labor and management can be expectant. PPROM often marks the onset of preterm labor and patients should be managed appropriately for their degree of prematurity. PPROM complicates approximately 30% of all preterm deliveries and is associated with significant morbidity and mortality. The most significant complication of PPROM is infection.

A number of factors have been associated with PROM including infectious, anatomic, and pregnancy-related factors (see Table 9.1). A considerable number of cases, however, are idiopathic. Trichomonas, bacterial vaginosis, urinary tract infection (UTI), gonorrhea, chlamydia, and group B strep are among the infectious agents known or suspected to be associated with PROM. Women with documented cervical incompetence are also at increased risk for PROM. Amniocentesis is associated with an increased risk of PROM. This risk may be, in part, related to the experience of the provider performing the procedure. For this reason, patients requiring amniocentesis should be referred to providers with considerable experience. Placental abruption is occasionally associated with PROM and should be considered in the evaluation of patients with PROM.

Diagnosis

History

Patients with PROM will often report discharge or "leaking" per vagina. This fluid leak may be subtle (e.g., increased wetness noted on undergarments or pants) or may be substantial (e.g., a "gush" of fluid). A careful history should be obtained to distinguish the causes of discharge such as cervical infection, physiological mucus production (or loss of the mucus plug), urinary incontinence, or UTI. Although each of these requires evaluation and diagnosis, management varies considerably from that for PROM.

Table 9.1 Risk factors for PROM

Infection
Hydramnios
Incompetent cervix
Placental abruption
Amniocentesis

Patients with PROM have, by definition, ruptured the membranes that serve to protect the infant from ascending infection. Patients with PROM are, therefore, at increased risk for perinatal transmission of genital infection and/or vaginal flora such as group B strep. This risk increases with the duration of rupture. For this reason, the best possible estimate of the time of rupture is an important part of the history. Because PROM represents the loss of protective membranes (and the subsequent risk of infection), every patient presenting with suggestive symptoms must be fully evaluated before eliminating PROM as a diagnosis.

Patients may also present with reported "urinary" symptoms such as urinary incontinence or urinary frequency. Such symptoms are both common and challenging. Anatomic changes associated with pregnancy such as increased uterine and fetal size increase urinary incontinence. Physiological changes associated with pregnancy such as relative outflow obstruction and urinary stasis increase the likelihood of urinary tract infection. For this reason, such urinary symptoms should be carefully detailed to identify other symptoms consistent with UTI such as urgency, dysuria, hematuria, abdominal pain, fever chills, nausea, vomiting, or back/costovertebral angle pain. As a general rule, evaluation of PROM should include assessment for UTI and evaluation of UTI should include assessment for PROM.

In addition to assessment for symptoms of urinary pathology, history should include information concerning bleeding per vagina and symptoms consistent with early or impending labor such as contractions, abdominal pain/cramps, back pain, or mucus plug loss. When symptoms that might be suggestive of more serious pathology are discovered, such as fever, bleeding, or severe pain, the history should be further expanded to include symptoms consistent with abruptio placenta, placenta previa, or infection/sepsis.

In addition to obtaining the history associated with the leakage of fluid, a brief review of the prenatal course is important. In particular, attention should be paid to prior infections, previous episodes of contractions or preterm labor, and prior episodes of bleeding or multiple gestations. Review of the gestational dating, the estimated date of delivery, and the data used to calculate these are also critical.

Physical Examination

If the history is consistent with possible PROM, providers should assume that the membranes have ruptured until this is ruled out. The primary concern under such circumstances is to minimize the possibility of ascending infection. Manual examinations should be minimized. Sterile speculum examination should be performed, and assessment should include testing for common infectious agents.

Vital signs should be documented and should include temperature, pulse, and blood pressure. A note should be made of patient discomfort or pain. Abdominal examination should include documentation of fundal height, abdominal tenderness,

Table 9.2 Leopold's maneuvers	First maneuver
	Identify fetal head, fetal body, and fundal height
	Second maneuver
	Palpate fetal body to determine position of the back (smooth and uninterrupted) and front (palpable fetal arms and legs)
	Third maneuver
	Move body side to side. Resistance to movement suggests fetal engagement
	Fourth maneuver
	Identify cephalic prominence

and fetal position (via Leopold's maneuvers; see Table 9.2). The external genitalia should be examined for evidence of infection (such as herpes), discharge, and trauma. On sterile speculum examination, note should be made of blood, fluid, or discharge in the vaginal vault or at the cervical os. Samples should be obtained for gonorrhea, chlamydia, group B strep, herpes (if characteristic or suspicious lesions are noted), yeast, and trichomonas/bacterial vaginosis.

Fetal heart rate should be documented including rate and variability. Uterine contractions should be noted on tocometer.

Laboratory

As noted previously, laboratory studies may include evaluation for gonorrhea, chlamydia, group B strep, herpes, trichomonas, and bacterial vaginosis. Although gonorrhea, chlamydia, group B strep, and herpes will not be immediately available, evaluation for yeast, trichomonas, and bacterial vaginosis can be performed quickly and accurately in the office. A microscopic examination of discharge/fluid may reveal clue cells (bacterial vaginosis), flagellated organisms (trichomonas), or fungal elements (yeast). A more comprehensive review of these conditions can be found in Chap. 13. A urine sample should be obtained for urinalysis, culture, and microscopic evaluation.

PROM is most accurately diagnosed via laboratory evidence of amniotic fluid in the vaginal vault. The two most common tests for rupture of membranes are nitrazine testing and "ferning." A sample of amniotic fluid placed on nitrazine paper will turn the paper blue. False positives may occur in the presence of blood, semen, or infection. A sample of the fluid should also be spread thinly on a microscope slide and allowed to air-dry. The dried sample should show characteristic fern-shaped crystalline pattern on microscopic examination.

Occasionally, suspected PROM may represent other more serious prenatal complications such as pyelonephritis, abruption, or pre-eclampsia. If these conditions are suspected on the basis of history or physical examination, additional laboratory studies will be necessary. Evaluation for these conditions should be reviewed in the appropriate chapters for each.

Management

The initial step in managing PROM is to distinguish PROM from PPROM. For this reason accurate gestational dating is critical. Figure 9.1 outlines the general management of PROM.

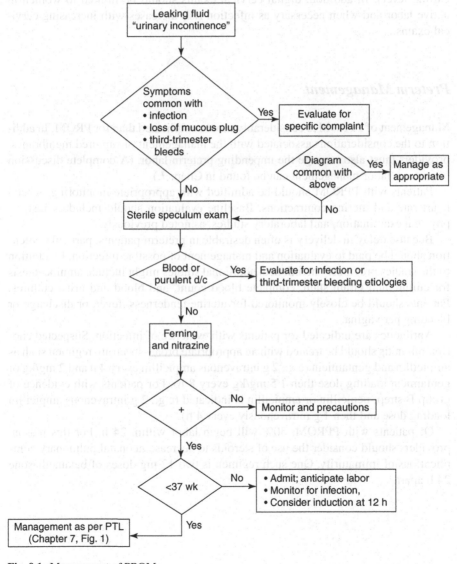

Fig. 9.1 Management of PROM

Management at Term

For patients determined to be at term (>37 weeks' gestation), management is similar to that for term labor. As the majority of these patients will begin labor within 24 h, no additional intervention will be necessary for many. Because the risk of infection increases as the duration of rupture increases, induction of labor may be necessary at 12 h or with signs/symptoms of fetal stress or infection (tachycardia, fetal tachycardia, fever). In addition, digital cervical exams should be limited to women in active labor and when necessary as infection risk increases with increasing cervical exams.

Preterm Management

Management of PPROM is considerably more complicated than for PROM. In addition to the considerations associated with the management of ruptured membranes, providers must also manage the impending preterm labor. (A complete discussion of preterm labor management can be found in Chap. 7.)

Patients with PPROM should be admitted with appropriate monitoring of fetal heart rate and uterine contractions. Baseline evaluation should include a history, physical examination, and laboratory studies, as noted previously.

Because delay in delivery is often desirable in preterm patients, particular attention should be paid to evaluation and management of possible infection. In addition to the studies previously mentioned, additional studies might include amniocentesis for culture and Gram stain, complete blood count, and blood and urine cultures. Patients should be closely monitored for uterine tenderness, fever, or discharge or bleeding per vagina.

Antibiotics are indicated for patients with evidence of infection. Suspected chorioamnionitis should be treated with an appropriate broad-spectrum regimen such as ampicillin and gentamicin (e.g., 2 g intravenous ampicillin every 4 h and 2 mg/kg of gentamicin loading dose then 1.5 mg/kg every 8 h). For patients with evidence of group B strep, penicillin or ampicillin is indicated (e.g., 2 g intravenous ampicillin loading dose and then 1 g intravenously every 4 h).

Of patients with PPROM, 50% will begin labor within 24 h. For this reason, providers should consider the use of steroids to decrease neonatal pulmonary complications of immaturity. One such regimen is two 12 mg doses of betamethasone 24 h apart.

Chapter 10
Early Pregnancy Bleeding

Contents

Background... 80
General Approach to Early Pregnancy Bleeding Per Vagina........................ 80
   History.. 81
   Physical Examination... 81
   Ultrasound.. 83
   Laboratory Studies.. 83
Ectopic Pregnancy... 84
   Background... 84
   Diagnosis... 84
   Management.. 85
   Surgical Management.. 86
   Medical Management.. 86
Spontaneous Abortion... 86
   Background... 86
   Diagnosis... 87
   Management.. 88

Key Points

1. Evaluation of early pregnancy bleeding should focus initially on identification of ectopic pregnancy and spontaneous abortion.
2. The primary concern of initial management is assessment of hemodynamic stability and possible peritonitis.
3. Management of ectopic pregnancy is designed to (a) minimize maternal morbidity and mortality, (b) remove the ectopic pregnancy, and (c) maximize potential future fertility.
4. Management of possible spontaneous abortion begins with ruling out the possibility of ectopic pregnancy.

© Springer Nature Switzerland AG 2020
P. Lyons, N. McLaughlin, *Obstetrics in Family Medicine*, Current Clinical Practice,
https://doi.org/10.1007/978-3-030-39888-0_10

Background

Bleeding per vagina may occur at any point during the course of pregnancy and always warrants careful attention to identification and management of the underlying etiology. Bleeding that occurs late in pregnancy (generally within the third trimester) is covered in Chap. 10. Bleeding that occurs early in pregnancy (generally within the first trimester) is of particular concern because of concerns with pregnancy viability and possible ectopic pregnancy with its associated morbidity and mortality. A careful review of common etiologies combined with a careful history, directed physical examination, and selected diagnostic studies will allow the provider to identify the underlying cause and initiate appropriate management in a timely manner.

Early pregnancy bleeding per vagina is a relatively common presentation, occurring in up to 25% of all pregnancies. Most cases of early bleeding are mild, self-limited, and of indeterminate etiology. Among the cases in which an etiology can be determined most are caused by either spontaneous abortion or ectopic pregnancy. Approximately 5–15% of all pregnancies will end in a clinically recognized spontaneous abortion (involuntary expulsion prior to 20 weeks' gestation). A considerably larger percentage (up to one-third) will end in an unrecognized abortion that is perceived to be menstrual bleeding. Although less common than spontaneous abortion, ectopic pregnancy is responsible for approximately 15% of all maternal deaths (6% in the United States). Although the differential diagnosis for early pregnancy bleeding includes several disparate conditions (*see* Table 10.1), the focus of initial evaluation is on identification of these two conditions. Less common causes of early pregnancy bleeding include trophoblastic disease and cervical pathology such as ulceration, infection, or cytopathology.

General Approach to Early Pregnancy Bleeding Per Vagina

As noted, most cases of early pregnancy bleeding per vagina are of indeterminate cause. A significant minority are related to spontaneous abortion. A smaller but significant number are associated with ectopic pregnancy. Initial evaluation will be directed toward identification of patients with these two conditions, documentation

Table 10.1 Conditions associated with early pregnancy bleeding

Ectopic pregnancy
Threatened abortion
Incomplete abortion
Complete abortion
Trophoblastic disease
Cervical polyps
Cervical ulceration
Cervical cytological abnormalities

of the viability of the pregnancy, assessment of the medical stability of the mother, and reassurance for patients without evidence of either condition. Figure 10.1 outlines a general approach to the evaluation and management of early pregnancy bleeding.

History

A careful history should be obtained of the bleeding itself as well as associated symptoms. In regard to the bleeding itself, information should be obtained concerning the following:

1. Characteristics of the bleeding (e.g., is it scant or copious, bright red or brown, and clot-like?).
2. Onset of the bleeding (e.g., did it start abruptly or gradually?).
3. Duration of the bleeding (how long has the bleeding lasted?).
4. Intensity of the bleeding (how much bleeding has been noticed? It may be helpful to use as comparison to normal menstrual flow, although providers should note that there is considerable physiological variability in the quantity of normal menstrual flow).
5. Exacerbating factors (did anything appear to precipitate the bleeding or make the bleeding worse once it had started?).
6. Relieving factors (has anything made the bleeding diminish or stop?).

Particular attention should be paid to trauma, activity (including sexual activity), and associated symptoms such as pain, dizziness, or weakness. The patient's past history should be reviewed for risk factors such as smoking, multiple sexual partners, past history of pelvic inflammatory disease, or intrauterine device use. Prior gynecological surgery should be reviewed, including tubal ligation and uterine surgery (including myomectomy). Any prior diagnosis of anatomic abnormalities of the genital tract should be noted. The patient's obstetrical history should be reviewed for prior ectopic pregnancies and/or spontaneous abortions. The prenatal course should be reviewed for any high-risk conditions that may have been previously noted, including a family history of significant genetic abnormalities or significant toxic or infectious exposures. A note should also be made of the patient's gestational age and the means used to determine the estimated delivery date.

Physical Examination

Physical examination begins with a rapid assessment of the hemodynamic stability of the mother. Depending on the gestational age of the patient, assessment of fetal heart rate may also be indicated. The mother's blood pressure (BP) and pulse should be

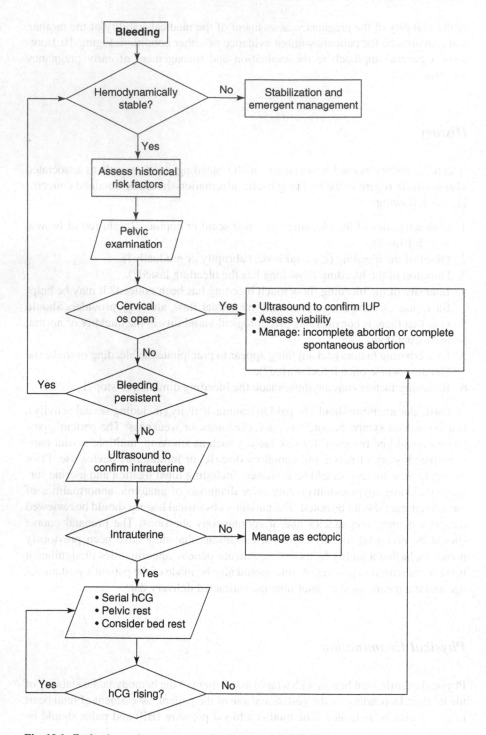

Fig. 10.1 Evaluation and management of early pregnancy bleeding

recorded including orthostatic measurements. (To measure orthostatic—positional—changes in BP and pulse, patients should first be placed in a recumbent position. BP and pulse are measured in the usual manner. The patient is then raised to a standing position and the pulse and BP are measured a second time. A note is made of a significant drop in BP or a significant rise in pulse.) The general assessment of the patient should include obvious signs of distress or discomfort. Abdominal examination should include assessment of uterine size. A pelvic examination should be performed. A note should be made of blood (location, at the cervical os, pooled in the vaginal vault; quantity: from scant discoloration to copious active bleeding; character, bright red, clotted, brown). Cervical status should be noted including dilation. The presence of other findings including discharge, amniotic fluid, or cervical lesions such as polyps or erosions should be documented. A bimanual examination should be performed to assess for adnexal mass or tenderness. The uterus should be assessed for size and tenderness.

Ultrasound

Ultrasound examination may be critical in the assessment of early pregnancy bleeding. Confirmation of an intrauterine pregnancy is possible as early as 5 weeks' gestation. In general, the presence of an intrauterine pregnancy significantly reduces *but does not eliminate* the possibility of ectopic pregnancy. Ultrasound examination is also diagnostic of trophoblastic disease. The absence of fetal heart activity may be indicative of a threatened or incomplete abortion. Transvaginal ultrasound is the study of choice for early pregnancy assessment. The absence of an intrauterine gestational sac after 6 weeks from the last menstrual period is strongly suggestive of nonviable pregnancy (ectopic or aborted). Transabdominal ultrasound may be used to assess for intra-abdominal fluid including blood.

Laboratory Studies

Early pregnancy bleeding per vagina may represent a significant obstetrical emergency in the case of an ectopic pregnancy that has ruptured. Blood loss may be rapid and difficult to control. For this reason, laboratory studies are ordered to establish baseline hematological status and in anticipation of a potential need for transfusion. Studies should include complete blood count with platelets, blood type, and cross-match. If not previously documented Rh status should be confirmed. The second key function of laboratory surveillance is to document the viability of the pregnancy. For this purpose, quantitative β-human chorionic gonadotropin (β-hCG) should be obtained.

Ectopic Pregnancy

Background

Ectopic pregnancy is diagnosed when pregnancy implantation occurs in a location outside the uterine cavity. The exact location can be variable and may include within the fallopian tubes (98%) or in an intraperitoneal/extrauterine location. Because blood supply and/or space is limited outside the uterine cavity, these pregnancies are capable of growing for a brief period but will eventually outgrow their space or blood supply. If the pregnancy implants in a location (such as the fallopian tube) where space is limited, rupture may occur with associated intraperitoneal bleeding.

Risk factors associated with an increased risk for ectopic pregnancy include prior history of ectopic pregnancy, prior history of pelvic inflammatory disease, prior pelvic surgery (including tubal ligation and reversal of tubal ligation), multiple sexual partners (probably related to an increased risk for unrecognized pelvic inflammatory disease and subsequent scarring), and smoking.

Diagnosis

History

Patients who present with early pregnancy bleeding per vagina should be carefully screened for risk factors that increase the probability of ectopic pregnancy as noted previously. Patients with ectopic pregnancy may report bleeding, abdominal pain, and symptoms of peritonitis, or it may be relatively asymptomatic. The bleeding may be variable depending on the location of the pregnancy. Although copious bleeding should prompt evaluation for ectopic pregnancy, providers should maintain a high index of suspicion as the absence of clinically apparent bleeding does not eliminate the possibility of ectopic pregnancy. The onset of symptoms may be acute but is often subacute with gradual worsening of symptoms that may be initially quite mild.

Physical Examination

The physical examination should include those elements noted previously to assess maternal and fetal well-being, including vital signs, abdominal examination, and fetal heart rate monitoring when appropriate. The physical examination may be quite variable. For some patients, the findings on physical examination are all normal. For others with rupture and significant intraperitoneal bleeding, findings may be indicative of acute peritonitis including diminished bowel sounds and a rigid, tender abdomen with rebound and guarding. A pelvic examination should be performed to assess for the presence of blood and/or products of conception, cervical status, uterine tenderness, adnexal tenderness, and adnexal mass.

Ultrasound Examination

Although history and physical examination may contribute to the diagnosis of ectopic pregnancy, all patients with early pregnancy bleeding per vagina should be assumed to have ectopic pregnancy until it is ruled out. For this reason, all patients should have ultrasound confirmation of the presence, viability, and location of the developing fetus. Ultrasound may demonstrate a gestational sac in the extrauterine space. Alternately, the ultrasound may show no evidence of a gestational sac despite elevated β-hCG levels. Transvaginal ultrasound should demonstrate intrauterine pregnancy when hCG levels reach approximately 6000 mIU/mL. Ectopic pregnancy should be strongly suspected if the ultrasound does not demonstrate either characteristic findings of trophoblastic disease or intrauterine pregnancy when β-hCG levels are greater than 2000 mIU/mL.

Laboratory Studies

Supportive laboratory studies include serum progesterone levels and serial quantitative β-hCG. Progesterone levels are rarely less than 5 ng/mL in viable pregnancies. Conversely, less than 1% of ectopic pregnancies will demonstrate serum progesterone levels of more than 25 ng/mL. Serum β-hCG may also add useful data. Ectopic pregnancy is rarely associated with β-hCG levels greater than 50,000 mIU/mL. If initial findings are equivocal, serial β-hCG levels are very helpful, so long as there is any rise in β-hCG level, continued monitoring is imperative. In normal pregnancies, serum β-hCG roughly doubles every 2–3 days. While there is variation depending on the starting β-hCG level, an increase in β-hCG less than 50% in 48 h is considered abnormal and should warrant further evaluation.

Management

Management of ectopic pregnancy depends considerably on the stability of the patient. Following diagnosis of ectopic pregnancy, patients should be assessed for clinical stability. Patients with hemodynamic instability or evidence of peritonitis should be considered surgical emergencies. For patients who are stable, evaluation for surgical or medical management may be performed. The purpose of management is threefold: (a) to minimize morbidity and mortality for the mother, (b) to remove the ectopic pregnancy, and (c) to maximize future potential fertility options.

In addition to the conditions just listed, indications for surgical intervention include anemia, gestational sac greater than 4 cm on ultrasound evaluation, pain of more than 24 h duration, suspected heterotopic pregnancy, or uncertainty of diagnosis requiring laparoscopic confirmation.

Indications for medical management include gestational sac smaller than 4 cm on ultrasound examination and hemodynamic stability.

Surgical Management

Patients with clinical evidence of hemodynamic instability or peritonitis should be treated as a surgical emergency. Providers should assume that blood products and fluid resuscitation will be necessary and should be prepared to provide both. Patients should be crossmatched for at least four units of blood and should have at least two large bore intravenous access sites established as quickly as possible. A variety of surgical options exist depending on the clinical presentation of the patient, the desire to preserve future fertility, and the experience of the operator. These options include salpingostomy, segmental resection, fimbrial expression, salpingectomy (in cases with significant bleeding, significant tubal damage, or recurrent ectopic pregnancies at the same location), and laparotomy (in cases with severe hemodynamic stability).

Medical Management

The use of methotrexate is a medical alternative to surgical management for appropriate patients. The success rate with single-dose methotrexate regimens is 80–90%. One such regimen is 50 mg/m^2 of methotrexate via intramuscular injection. Serum β-hCG levels are obtained on days 1, 4, and 7. A second dose is administered on day 7 if serum β-hCG has not demonstrated a significant (~15%) decrease. Serial weekly serum β-hCG levels should be obtained until levels are less than 15 mIU/mL.

Spontaneous Abortion

Background

Among cases of early pregnancy bleeding with a known etiology, spontaneous abortion is by far the most common. As noted, 5–15% of all pregnancies will end with a clinically apparent spontaneous abortion; up to one-third of all pregnancies end in spontaneous abortion. Although generally spontaneous abortion is not as medically concerning as ectopic pregnancy, the significance of spontaneous abortion for the patient (and her family) will often be quite high. For this reason, appropriate diagnosis and management of spontaneous abortion is critical.

Risk factors for spontaneous abortion include genetic abnormalities, toxic exposures, structural abnormalities (such as atypical uterine anatomy), smoking, and toxic exposure. Most cases of spontaneous abortion occur without a clinically apparent risk factor.

Spontaneous abortion may be divided into three general subtypes: threatened, incomplete, and complete.

Threatened abortion is defined as bleeding per vagina before 20 weeks without passage of tissue or premature rupture of membranes. Threatened abortion may present with or without cervical dilation. Bleeding per vagina prior to 20 weeks' gestation in conjunction with cervical dilation is referred to as inevitable abortion.

Incomplete abortion is defined as bleeding and incomplete passage of the products of conception. This condition may be associated with hemodynamic instability in which case it should be considered an obstetrical emergency and should include all the usual elements associated with management of such unstable patients.

Complete abortion is defined as bleeding with complete passage of all products of conception. The distinction between incomplete and complete abortion is not always clear, and care should be exercised to confirm the passage of all products prior to making the diagnosis of complete abortion.

Diagnosis

It should be recognized that patients will not present with a chief complaint of spontaneous abortion; they will present with a complaint of bleeding per vagina. For this reason, the general history for these patients will mirror that of patients with ectopic pregnancy.

History

History should include the elements described earlier, including a history of the bleeding, associated symptoms, a review of historical risk factors, and symptoms of hemodynamic instability. Particular attention should be paid to reports of passage of tissue or "clots." A past history of spontaneous abortion should raise providers' suspicion of abortion.

Physical Examination

Physical examination will begin with assessment of the hemodynamic stability of the patient. Pelvic examination will assess cervical dilation, bleeding, and/or products of conception. To assess for other potential causes of bleeding, providers should make note of adnexal tenderness or mass, cervical lesions, discharge, or other abnormalities.

Ultrasound Examination

The use of ultrasound in suspected abortion may provide limited but useful information. Ultrasound examination may demonstrate the presence or absence of a gestational sac, the presence or absence of fetal cardiac activity, and the evidence of retained products of conception.

Laboratory Studies

Laboratory studies are generally limited for patients who are clinically stable. Serial serum β-hCG levels should be obtained to document continued viability (for threatened abortion) or appropriate decline in levels (incomplete or complete abortion). For patients who are clinically unstable, laboratory studies are the same as noted for ectopic pregnancy.

Management

Threatened Abortion

Effective management of threatened abortion is quite limited. Bedrest does not improve outcomes in threatened abortion and the use of progesterone lacks sufficient evidence for use. As noted earlier, documentation of serum β-hCG levels may be helpful.

Incomplete Abortion

By definition, patients with incomplete abortion no longer have a viable pregnancy and have not yet passed all of the products of conception. Management requires (a) assessment of hemodynamic stability, (b) removal of retained products of conception, and (c) documentation of declining serum β-hCG levels to confirm adequacy of treatment. For hemodynamically unstable patients, management includes fluids, blood, and rapid surgical intervention. The use of oxytocin (30–40 U/L of fluid) may help control bleeding. For stable patients, surgical evacuation should be performed and serial serum β-hCG levels obtained. Patients who are Rh negative should receive rhogam at the time of dilation and evacuation to prevent isoimmunization.

Complete Abortion

Management of patients with confirmed complete abortion is relatively straightforward. No intervention is required and serial serum β-hCG levels should be sufficient to document adequacy of management. As previously noted, however, providers should exercise caution as the distinction between complete and incomplete abortions is not always clinically apparent.

Chapter 11
Late-Pregnancy Bleeding

Contents

Background... 92
General Approach to Late-Pregnancy Bleeding Per Vagina.................... 92
   History.. 94
   Ultrasound.. 94
   Physical Examination.. 95
   Laboratory Studies.. 95
Placenta Previa.. 95
   Background.. 95
   History... 96
   Ultrasound Examination.. 96
   Physical Examination.. 96
   Laboratory Studies.. 96
   Management.. 97
   Management at Term.. 97
   Preterm Management.. 97
Abruptio Placenta.. 97
   Background.. 97
   History... 98
   Ultrasound.. 98
   Physical Examination.. 98
   Laboratory Studies.. 99
   Management.. 99
   Management of Mild Abruption.. 99
   Management of Moderate or Severe Abruption.............................. 99

> **Key Points**
> 1. Initial assessment of late-pregnancy bleeding is designed to identify potential placenta previa and abruptio placentae.
> 2. No manual or speculum examination should be performed until placenta previa has been ruled out.

© Springer Nature Switzerland AG 2020
P. Lyons, N. McLaughlin, *Obstetrics in Family Medicine*, Current Clinical Practice,
https://doi.org/10.1007/978-3-030-39888-0_11

3. Placenta previa is an absolute contraindication to vaginal delivery.
4. Placenta previa and abruptio placentae are obstetrical emergencies and require rapid assessment and management.
5. Initial management of placenta previa and abruptio placentae is directed toward ensuring hemodynamic stability and safe delivery.

Background

Bleeding per vagina may occur at any point during the course of pregnancy and always warrants careful attention to identification and management of the underlying etiology. Bleeding that occurs early in pregnancy (generally within the first trimester) is covered in Chap. 9. Bleeding that occurs later in pregnancy (generally within the third trimester) is of particular concern because of the potentially serious underlying etiologies and the possibility of significant morbidity that exists for both the mother and the infant. A careful review of common etiologies combined with a careful history, directed physical examination, and selected diagnostic studies will allow the provider to identify the underlying cause and initiate appropriate management in a timely manner.

Late-pregnancy bleeding per vagina is a relatively common presentation. Approximately 5% of all pregnancies is complicated by such bleeding. Although the differential diagnosis includes several disparate conditions, placental abnormalities comprise the majority of such bleeding (*see* Table 11.1). Half of all third-trimester bleeding is caused by either placental abruption or placenta previa. Vasa previa is a much less common, but still potentially devastating, cause of late pregnancy bleeding. Other causes include cervical cytopathology, polyps, and "bloody show." Bloody show refers to limited bleeding per vagina just prior to or at the onset of labor. Such bleeding is a variant of normal, although patients may require evaluation for other causes of bleeding.

General Approach to Late-Pregnancy Bleeding Per Vagina

Most cases of significant late-pregnancy bleeding per vagina are caused by placental abnormalities: placental abruption and placenta previa. The diagnosis and man-

Table 11.1 Conditions associated with late-pregnancy bleeding

Placenta previa
Placental abruption
Vasa previa
Cervical cytopathology
Polyps
"Bloody show"

agement of each is detailed here. When faced with a patient who presents with bleeding per vagina, however, a general approach to evaluation (outlined in Fig. 11.1) will allow for rapid evaluation and triage of those patients with such significant obstetrical problems from those with other less common presentations.

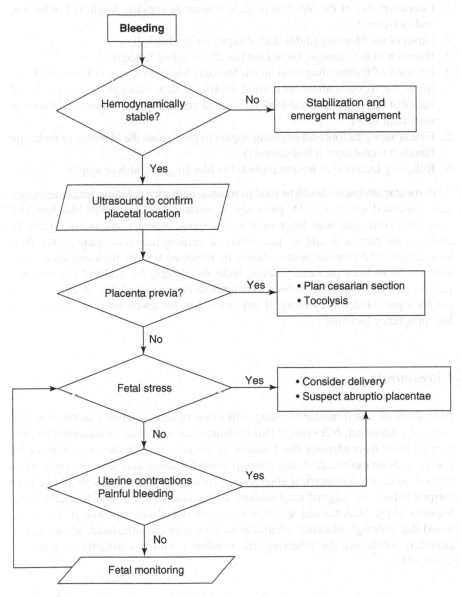

Fig. 11.1 Management of late-pregnancy bleeding

History

A careful history should be obtained of the bleeding itself as well as associated symptoms. In regard to the bleeding itself, information should be obtained concerning the following:

1. Characteristics of the bleeding (e.g., is it scant or copious, bright red or brown, and clot-like?)
2. Onset of the bleeding (did it start abruptly or gradually?)
3. Duration of the bleeding (how long has the bleeding lasted?)
4. Intensity of the bleeding (how much bleeding has been noticed? It may be helpful to use as comparison to normal menstrual flow although providers should note that there is considerable physiological variability in the quantity of normal menstrual flow)
5. Exacerbating factors (did anything appear to precipitate the bleeding or make the bleeding worse once it had started?)
6. Relieving factors (has anything made the bleeding diminish or stop?)

Particular attention should be paid to trauma, activity (including sexual activity), and associated symptoms. Of particular importance are pain with bleeding and symptoms consistent with labor such as cramping, contractions, or back pain. In addition, the patient should be questioned concerning fetal movement and/or fetal kick counts. The prenatal course should be reviewed for any high-risk conditions that may have been previously noted. Note should also be made of the patient's gestational age and the means used to determine the estimated date of delivery. The patient's past obstetrical history, if any, should be reviewed for prior episodes of late-pregnancy bleeding.

Ultrasound

Evaluation of late trimester bleeding will often require a pelvic examination and cervical assessment. *It is critical that no manual or speculum examination be performed prior to confirming the location of the placenta.* In the case of placenta previa, such an examination may cause placental damage and acute severe hemorrhage leading to an obstetrical emergency. Ultrasound examination should be performed before any vaginal examination. Ultrasound may be used to identify the location of the placenta and specifically to rule out placenta previa. It should be noted that although placental abruption *may* be seen on ultrasound, ultrasound is generally ineffective for detecting this condition with a sensitivity of approximately 15%.

Physical Examination

Physical examination begins with a rapid assessment of the hemodynamic stability of the mother and of the fetal well-being. The mother's blood pressure and pulse should be recorded. The patient should be placed on electronic monitoring to assess fetal heart rate and contractions, if any. The general assessment of the patient should include obvious signs of distress or discomfort. Abdominal examination should include assessment of fetal size and position. Following ultrasound examination to determine the placental position, a pelvic examination should be performed. Note should be made of blood (location, at the cervical os, pooled in the vaginal vault; quantity, from scant discoloration to copious active bleeding; character, bright red, clotted, brown). Cervical status should be noted, including dilation and effacement. The presence of other findings, including discharge, amniotic fluid, or cervical lesions such as polyps or erosions, should be documented. The position of the fetus should be confirmed, including presenting part and station. The uterus should be assessed for size and tenderness.

Laboratory Studies

Late-pregnancy bleeding per vagina may represent a significant obstetrical emergency. Blood loss may be rapid and difficult to control. For this reason, laboratory studies are ordered to establish baseline hematological status and in anticipation of a potential need for transfusion. Studies should include complete blood count with platelets, international normalized ratio, partial thromboplastin time, fibrinogen, fibrin split products, blood type, and crossmatch.

Placenta Previa

Background

Placenta previa may be diagnosed when the placenta is located in such a position as to partially or completely occlude the internal cervical os (and therefore to occlude the outflow tract of the birth canal). Total or complete placenta previa, as the name implies, represents occlusion of the entire cervical os. Partial placenta previa represents less than complete occlusion. A marginal placenta signifies a location adjacent to but not occluding the cervical os. Although these categories are useful guides, it should be noted that the distinction may not be entirely clear on ultrasound examination. For this reason, particular caution should be exercised whenever the location of the placenta appears to be near or over the cervical os.

Under such circumstances, cervical dilation and/or direct trauma (such as fetal descent or pelvic examination) may cause laceration of the placenta and subsequent bleeding. Because of the highly vascular nature of the placenta, such bleeding may be rapid, copious, and life-threatening to both the mother and the fetus. Placental previa is estimated to occur in approximately 1 out of every 100 pregnancies.

History

Patients who present with late-pregnancy bleeding per vagina should be carefully screened for risk factors that increase the probability of placenta previa. These risk factors include prior dilation and curettage, myomectomy, cesarean section, maternal age (prevalence increases with increasing maternal age), grand multiparity, and multiple gestation. The primary symptom associated with placenta previa is bleeding per vagina. The onset is usually acute, may be associated with trauma or physical manipulation such as examination, is often continuous, and may be variable but can be significant. It is classically not associated with pain (although the presence of pain *does not* rule out the possibility of placenta previa).

Ultrasound Examination

Although these historical factors may contribute to the diagnosis of placenta previa, all patients with late-pregnancy bleeding per vagina should be assumed to have placenta previa until it is ruled out. For this reason, all patients should have ultrasound confirmation of the location of the placenta prior to manual or speculum examination. If prior ultrasound examinations have demonstrated a placental location away from the cervical os, this is sufficient to rule out placenta previa as the placenta may migrate away from the cervical os but does not migrate toward the cervical os.

Physical Examination

The physical examination should include those elements noted previously to assess maternal and fetal well-being, including vital signs, abdominal examination, fetal heart rate monitoring, and monitoring for contractions. For patients in whom the ultrasound confirms placenta previa, no manual or speculum examination should be performed.

Laboratory Studies

Laboratory studies are the same as those noted previously.

Management

Providers should assume that blood products and fluid resuscitation will be necessary and be prepared to provide both. Patients with confirmed placenta previa should be crossmatched for at least four units of blood and should have at least two large bore intravenous access sites established as quickly as possible. If the patient is actively contracting, tocolysis may be indicated to lessen the risk of further placental damage and bleeding.

Management at Term

For patients who have reached at least 36 weeks' gestation, cesarean section is indicated. Placenta previa is an absolute contraindication to vaginal delivery. If the patient is actively contracting and the cesarean section cannot be performed immediately, tocolysis is indicated. Delivery of the infant and the placenta is the definitive treatment for placenta previa. Patients should be monitored for hemodynamic stability with blood and/or fluids administered to maintain adequate blood pressure and to replete circulating blood volume.

Preterm Management

Placenta previa with active bleeding per vagina is an obstetrical emergency. If the mother or infant is unstable and/or the bleeding cannot be controlled, cesarean section is indicated. Management of maternal hemodynamic status is the same as at term. Neonatal specialists should be present at the delivery to manage the newborn. For preterm patients who are stable and not bleeding, care should be individualized. Such care might include tocolysis, assessment of fetal lung maturity, and preparation for cesarean section.

Abruptio Placenta

Background

The maintenance of fetal perfusion, oxygenation, and nutrition requires the maintenance of the maternal–fetal placental unit. The interruption of placental function secondary to separation of the placental from the uterine wall is referred to as abruptio placenta or placental abruption. As with placenta previa, the severity of the condition may vary from minor separation with minimal signs or symptoms to complete abruption with significant compromise of maternal and/or fetal well-being. Although the variability in presentation makes exact prevalence difficult to calculate, it is estimated that 1 out of 100 pregnancies are affected by significant placental abruption.

The classic presentation for placental abruption is abrupt onset painful bleeding with associated uterine contractions. However, the variability in severity as well as location of the abruption makes such "classic" presentations rather uncommon. Up to 80% of all cases of placental abruption present with no clinically apparent bleeding. The severity of the condition cannot be reliably predicted based on the quantity of clinically apparent bleeding. Patients with known or suspected placental abruption should be assumed to have bled significantly until proven otherwise. Because of the variability in presentation, providers should have a low threshold for suspecting placental abruption and manage such patients diligently.

History

As noted, the classic presentation for placental abruption is late-pregnancy bleeding per vagina. The bleeding is associated with abdominal or back pain, acute in onset, and variable in quantity (or perhaps absent). Patients will often report the acute onset (or an acute increase in severity) of uterine contractions.

Ultrasound

As with all patients with late-pregnancy bleeding per vagina, no pelvic examination should be performed until ultrasound confirmation of placental location has been obtained. Although ultrasound has a very low sensitivity for detection of placental abruption, approximately 15% of cases are ultrasonographically apparent.

Physical Examination

In general, the physical examination does not contribute significantly to the diagnosis of placental abruption. Suggestive findings include hemodynamic instability, evidence of fetal stress on fetal heart rate monitoring, firm or tender uterus, and/or back tenderness. Although neither sensitive nor specific, the finding of a very firm uterus that does not relax (or hypertonic uterus on tocometer) should prompt immediate consideration of the possibility of placental abruption. All patients with suspected abruption should be placed on fetal heart rate monitoring, tocometer, and hemodynamic monitoring, including blood pressure and pulse.

Laboratory Studies

Laboratory studies are as noted in the previous sections.

Management

Appropriate management depends on a clinical assessment of the severity of the condition. As noted, however, the physical findings associated with abruption may be highly variable. When doubt exists concerning the severity of the condition, it is advisable to make preparations for management of severe abruption with significant maternal or fetal compromise.

Management of Mild Abruption

If the bleeding is mild or absent and both mother and fetus are clinically stable, management can be expectant. Patients should be placed on continuous hemodynamic, fetal heart rate and uterine contraction monitoring. Evidence of stability includes normal maternal blood pressure and pulse and minimal symptoms. Fetal heart rate monitoring should demonstrate normal heart rate with adequate variability. Uterine contraction pattern should be monitored for signs of hypertonicity or tetanus. If the patient is preterm, tocolysis may be indicated to facilitate fetal lung maturity. Maternal coagulation status should also be monitored. Because of the possibility of worsening abruption and hemodynamic instability, all patients should have at least two large bore intravenous access sites and should have adequate cross-matched blood available.

Management of Moderate or Severe Abruption

For patients with more significant clinical abruption, management must focus on two primary concerns: management of the hemodynamic status of the mother and rapid delivery of the infant. Maternal shock and/or disseminated intravascular coagulation are possible sequela of severe placental abruption. These patients will require emergent management with particular attention to the "ABCs" (airway, breathing, circulation) as dictated by the clinical presentation. Patients may require fluid infusion and/or blood product transfusion that may include fresh frozen plasma, cryoprecipitate, or platelets.

A clinical decision must be made concerning the instability of the mother and the likelihood of delivery. In less severe cases, induction of labor may be appropriate. In more severe cases, cesarean section may be indicated for more rapid delivery of the infant. Neonatology support should be present at the time of delivery for management of the newborn.

Chapter 12
Recurrent Pregnancy Loss

Contents

Background.. 101
Diagnosis... 103
Management.. 103
   History... 103
   Physical Examination... 104
   Diagnostic Studies.. 104

> **Key Points**
> 1. Spontaneous abortion is defined as delivery prior to 20 weeks' gestation.
> 2. Recurrent pregnancy loss is defined as three or more spontaneous abortions prior to 20 weeks' gestation.
> 3. Limited but consistent data suggests that the use of progesterone is associated with decreased rate of recurrent pregnancy loss and preterm labor as well as increased rate of live birth

Background

Spontaneous abortion is a common outcome of pregnancy, especially in the first trimester of pregnancy. Defined as delivery prior to 20 weeks of gestation, spontaneous abortion is often an unexpected and traumatic experience for the patient and her family. Spontaneous abortion is discussed in detail in Chap. 9. Briefly, abortion can be considered to fall into one of two categories: complete abortion, which is defined as delivery of all products of conception prior to 20 weeks' gestation, or incomplete abortion, defined as delivery of some but not all products of conception prior to 20 weeks' gestation.

P. Lyons, N. McLaughlin, *Obstetrics in Family Medicine*, Current Clinical Practice,
https://doi.org/10.1007/978-3-030-39888-0_12

In addition to these two categories, first-trimester bleeding can also indicate a possible impending abortion. Uterine bleeding prior to 20 weeks' gestation without delivery of any products of conception is considered a threatened abortion. Uterine bleeding prior to 20 weeks with cervical dilation but without delivery of products of conception is referred to as an inevitable abortion.

Although spontaneous abortion is common, recurrent pregnancy loss (three or more consecutive abortions prior to 20 weeks' delivery) is considerably less common, affecting approximately 1% of all women of childbearing age. In addition to the evaluation and management considerations that pertain to a single episode of spontaneous abortion, recurrent spontaneous abortions require further evaluation and more significant management considerations (see Table 12.1).

Prior spontaneous abortion increases the risk for subsequent abortion, although the degree of risk is not well quantified. As noted in Chap. 10, spontaneous abortion, often not clinically diagnosed, occurs in up to one-third of all pregnancies. Among patients with a history of spontaneous abortion, the risk of spontaneous abortion rises to approximately 30% after two prior spontaneous abortions and to approximately 50% after three prior episodes. Although that makes recurrence a frequent event, it should be emphasized that it is by no means inevitable.

Table 12.1 Risk factors for recurrent pregnancy loss

Exogenous exposures
Alcohol
Tobacco
Cocaine
Obstetrical/gynecological abnormalities
Uterine abnormalities
Leiomyomas
Genetic uterine anatomic abnormalities (bicornuate, septate)
Cervical incompetence
Diethylstilbestrol exposure
Asherman's syndrome
Infection (gonorrhea, chlamydia, syphilis, listeria, mycoplasma, ureaplasma, toxoplasma)
Progesterone deficiency
Genetic abnormalities
Chronic medical conditions
Thyroid disease (hypothyroid and hyperthyroid)
Renal disease
Uncontrolled diabetes mellitus
Collagen vascular disease
Uncontrolled hypertension
Antiphospholipid antibodies (anticardiolipin antibody, lupus anticoagulant)

Diagnosis

The diagnosis of recurrent spontaneous abortion is made clinically in patients with an appropriate history. Although additional evaluation may be appropriate for evaluation and management purposes, no additional studies are required to make the diagnosis.

Management

Management of recurrent spontaneous abortion begins with a careful history, a directed physical examination, and diagnostic studies to elucidate an etiology. Although not all cases of recurrent spontaneous abortion will have an identified cause, identification of such a cause when present may contribute to successful management. In general, identified causes will fall into the categories of exogenous exposures (such as medication, tobacco, alcohol, illicit drugs, and occupational exposures), obstetrical or gynecological abnormalities, genetic abnormalities, or chronic medical conditions (such as renal disease, and diabetes). In general, outcomes for patients with recurrent abortions are good, with at least half of such patients eventually carrying a pregnancy to term.

History

A careful history should be obtained. The history should focus on likely underlying causes. As would be expected, the history begins with a focus on prior obstetrical and gynecological conditions. All previous pregnancies should be reviewed for complications and outcomes. Abnormal menstrual cycles may be indicative of hormonal dysregulation or previously unrecognized spontaneous abortions. Gynecological history should focus on fertility, especially hypofertility, and any known anatomic abnormalities. Gynecological surgeries, especially those involving the cervix, should be reviewed. A past history of sexually transmitted disease (STD) should be obtained as well as a history of any current symptoms consistent with STD.

The patient's exposure to exogenous agents should include medications, occupational exposures, and tobacco, alcohol, or illicit drug use. All medications, including over-the-counter, prescription, and complementary/alternative modalities, should be reviewed. If the provider is unfamiliar with any of the medications, referral to a maternal–fetal medicine specialist might be considered. The patient's work history should be reviewed for possible occupational exposures. Although less common as a source of exogenous toxins, the patient's hobbies and recreational activities should also be reviewed.

A review of the patient's family history may be helpful in at least two regards. A careful genogram for possible genetic abnormalities should be obtained. A genetics counselor may provide assistance with obtaining this history and the genogram. Additionally, the family history may reveal a familial predisposition to a variety of medical conditions for which the patient is at risk. Hypertension, diabetes, renal disease, and coagulopathies, among other disease processes, may be familial and may contribute to an increased risk for spontaneous.

Physical Examination

The physical examination is often directed by the findings of the history and is more limited in scope. The patient's vital signs, particularly her blood pressure, should be measured. Examination of the head/neck should include palpation of the thyroid for enlargement and/or nodularity. Additionally, examination of the eyes may reveal evidence of hypertensive or diabetic retinal changes. Examination of the skin should be performed to detect the physical stigmata of endocrine disorders such as striae or changes in skin texture, consistency, or color. Cardiovascular examination should include documentation of murmurs, if any (especially renal bruits), and peripheral pulses. Neurological examination should include documentation of the peripheral sensory function.

Although unlikely to demonstrate any abnormalities, a pelvic examination should be performed to document normal anatomy and to obtain cervical samples for gonococcus and chlamydia.

Diagnostic Studies

Diagnostic studies will be directed toward the common underlying etiologies for recurrent spontaneous abortion. If genetic causes are suspected, these studies include karyotyping of both parents. Routine laboratory studies include cervical sampling for gonorrhea/chlamydia, progesterone, thyroid-stimulating hormone, thyroxine, lupus anticoagulant, and anticardiolipin antibody. If diabetes is suspected on the basis of family history or patient symptoms, a fasting blood sugar may help to clarify the diagnosis. Renal function may be assessed via routine blood serum electrolyte testing and urinalysis. Under limited circumstances, a serum drug screen may be indicated, although this diagnosis is generally made by history rather than by laboratory studies. If anatomic abnormalities are suspected, evaluation of the lower reproductive tract via radiological (hysterosalpingogram, pelvic ultrasound) or endoscopic (hysteroscopy) means is indicated.

Management of subsequent pregnancies will depend in large measure on the findings of this diagnostic evaluation. Although several of the identified conditions are not directly correctable, others are. Treatment of infection, management of hypertension, treatment of thyroid disease, and elimination or reduction of toxic exposures may all enhance the likelihood of a successful pregnancy.

Only half of patients with recurrent spontaneous abortion will have an identified cause. For patients in whom no definitive cause is identified, the use of progestin in early pregnancy has been suggested. Review data suggests limited but consistent data that the use of progestin is associated with a decreased rate of recurrent abortion and preterm labor. It is also associated with an increased rate of live birth. The use of progestin is supported only early in the course of pregnancy. No evidence exists to support its use as a rescue agent once evidence of spontaneous abortion is noted. Many patients with recurrent pregnancy loss will be managed in conjunction with a provider who specializes in this area of obstetrics.

Chapter 13
Rh Isoimmunization

Contents

Background... 107
Fetal Consequences of Isoimmunization... 108
Newborn Consequences of Isoimmunization.. 109
Diagnosis.. 109
   History... 109
   Physical Examination.. 109
   Diagnostic Studies.. 109
Management Prior to Isoimmunization.. 110
Management of Pregnancies with Rh-Sensitized Mothers............................. 110
   Amniotic Fluid Assessment.. 112
   Ultrasonography.. 112
   Percutaneous Umbilical Blood Sampling.. 112

> **Key Points**
> 1. Rh isoimmunization represents a maternal antibody response to immuno-logically incompatible fetal blood.
> 2. Rh isoimmunization is a preventable outcome of maternal–fetal Rh incompatibility.
> 3. Fetal blood should be considered Rh positive unless documented otherwise.

Background

Transfer of nutrients, proteins, and antibodies between the mother and fetus gener-ally occurs across the placenta without direct transfer of blood. Although the mater-nal and fetal blood supplies are separated from each other, they are, of necessity, in relative proximity and can, under certain circumstances, come into contact with

© Springer Nature Switzerland AG 2020

P. Lyons, N. McLaughlin, *Obstetrics in Family Medicine*, Current Clinical Practice,
https://doi.org/10.1007/978-3-030-39888-0_13

each other. Under these circumstances, exposure to foreign proteins may elicit an immune response with potential health effects for either the mother or fetus.

Rh isoimmunization represents a serious maternal–fetal complication. All red blood cells are produced with a variety of surface antibodies that serve to identify one's own red cells from those of others. The presence of red blood cells from an outside source will elicit an immune response with subsequent hemolysis/removal of the foreign cells. This response may be relatively minor or may represent a significant medical complication.

The primary surface proteins serve to identify blood within the ABO blood type categories. Exposure to immunologically incompatible blood types within the ABO category will result in significant hematological complications. A second set of proteins (rhesus factor) also provide significant identification. Rh-negative ([Rh−] those without Rh factor) patients exposed to blood containing Rh factor (Rh positive [Rh+]) will produce an antibody response to that blood. It is this incompatibility that results in the complications of Rh isoimmunization. An initial exposure will lead to development of antibodies. Subsequent exposures will yield a significant antibody response and an associated reaction.

Pregnant Rh-negative patients exposed to fetal Rh-positive blood may also develop such an antibody response (approximately 20% will isoimmunize if not treated). Because such antibodies can cross the placenta and reach the fetus, all subsequent pregnancies that involve Rh-positive fetuses will potentially result in hemolysis and in complications for the fetus.

Rh factor is a genetically inherited trait with an autosomal-dominant inheritance pattern. An Rh-negative mother is, by definition, homozygous (Rh−/Rh−). An Rh-positive father may be homozygous (Rh+/Rh+) or heterozygous (Rh+/Rh−). As all children will receive one Rh-negative gene from such mothers, the Rh status of the child is dependent on the Rh status of the father. All children of homozygous Rh-positive fathers will be Rh positive. One-half of all children of heterozygous fathers will be Rh positive.

Fetal Consequences of Isoimmunization

Although maternal blood does not generally cross the placenta, maternal antibodies do. The placental transmission of maternal antibodies to Rh factor will result in fetal hemolysis and subsequent anemia. In addition, the red blood cell destruction results in the release of heme and bilirubin. These breakdown products are cleared by the maternal circulation after crossing the placenta. The results for the fetus are generally related to complications of severe anemia (erythroblastosis fetalis) and may include heart failure, acute pericardial effusion, hypoxia, acidosis, and death.

Newborn Consequences of Isoimmunization

Following delivery, Rh-isoimmunized infants lose access to the maternal circulation but will continue to have circulating maternal antibodies. Under these circumstances, the neonate may be incapable of adequately clearing the bilirubin and heme that result from continued red blood cell destruction. The potential complications for infants will include those anemia, cardiac complications, acidosis, and death, as well as deposition of heme within the basal ganglia of the developing brain (kernicterus).

Diagnosis

History

The Rh status of the infant is usually unknown; therefore, particular care should be taken to note the Rh status of the mother. When known, the Rh status of the father should also be noted. Prior pregnancies should be recorded, including the Rh status of the resulting infant. If the patient has had prior pregnancies, any administration of Rh immunoglobulin (discussed later) should be recorded. As noted previously, the initial exposure is less significant than subsequent exposures. For this reason, the history is particularly important in second and subsequent pregnancies.

Physical Examination

In general, the physical examination will not contribute to the diagnosis of Rh iso-immunization, but careful monitoring of fetal growth and development is critical in the management of pregnancies complicated by Rh isoimmunization.

Diagnostic Studies

Rh factor should be documented for all pregnant patients. For those patients found to be Rh negative, paternal testing may be indicated. If paternity is uncertain or paternal testing cannot be performed, the infants should be assumed to be Rh positive and management should proceed accordingly.

Management Prior to Isoimmunization

Overall management of Rh− patients is outlined in Fig. 13.1. The management of pregnancies with the potential for isoimmunization consists of the following three key principles:

1. Minimize the potential for maternal–fetal transfusion (*see* Table 13.1).
2. Administer Rh immunoglobulin if maternal–fetal transfusion is known or suspected.
3. Because all pregnancies are potentially complicated by minor maternal–fetal transfusions not recognizable clinically, all Rh-negative patients will receive immunoglobulin at about 28 weeks' gestation.

At 28 weeks' gestation, Rh-negative patients should be tested for evidence of Rh antibodies. If no antibodies are detected, patients should receive 300 μg of Rh immunoglobulin as a single intramuscular dose. Following delivery, the Rh status of the infant should be determined. If the infant is found to be Rh positive, a second dose of Rh immunoglobulin should be administered within the first 72 h postpartum.

Under all circumstances where maternal–fetal transfusion is possible or suspected, patients should receive Rh immunoglobulin. In general, a single dose is sufficient for most exposures. If a larger-than-usual transfusion is suspected, further testing should be performed to determine the extent of exposure and additional doses of immunoglobulin may be necessary. This occurs in less than 1 out of 200 cases.

Management of Pregnancies with Rh-Sensitized Mothers

Management of the first pregnancy associated with isoimmunization is generally uncomplicated and will follow the guidelines for usual pregnancy management. Infants may require additional monitoring postpartum but can be expected to follow the usual newborn course. All Rh-sensitized mothers, however, should be informed of the development, the nature of the problem, and its potential effects in subsequent pregnancies. Critical discussions of contraception, preconception counseling, and future pregnancy planning should begin in the immediate postpartum period.

Patients known to be previously Rh sensitized require careful management and involvement of a skilled maternal–fetal medicine provider. Although a full discussion of the management of such patients is beyond the scope of this text, the general course of management is reviewed here.

For previously sensitized patients, antibody titers should be drawn at intake, at 20 weeks' gestation, and every 4 weeks thereafter. If antibody titers remain below 1:8, careful antenatal monitoring and continued routine prenatal care are recommended. When titers rise above a critical threshold (1:8–1:32), management will proceed as described below.

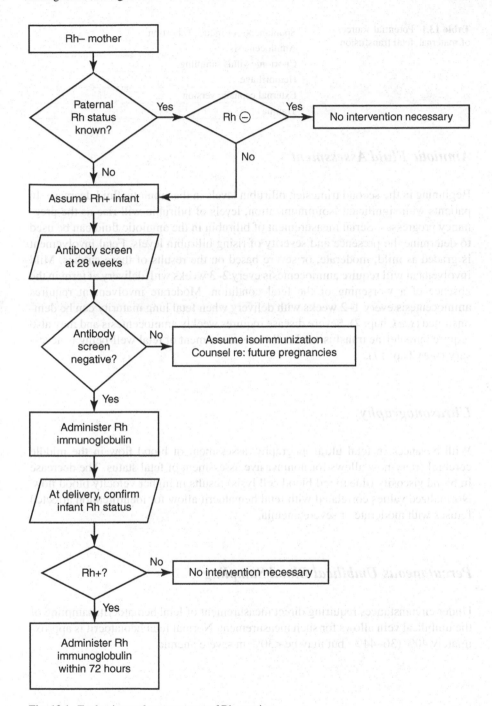

Fig. 13.1 Evaluation and management of Rh− patient

Table 13.1 Potential sources
of maternal–fetal transfusion

Spontaneous or induced abortion
Amniocentesis
Chorionic villus sampling
Hemorrhage
External cephalic version
Trauma

Amniotic Fluid Assessment

Beginning in the second trimester, bilirubin levels in the amniotic fluid decrease. In patients with significant isoimmunization, levels of bilirubin will rise as the pregnancy progresses. Serial measurement of bilirubin in the amniotic fluid can be used to determine the presence and severity of rising bilirubin levels. Fetal involvement is graded as mild, moderate, or severe based on the results of these studies. Mild involvement will require amniocentesis every 2–3 weeks with delivery at term in the absence of a worsening of the fetal condition. Moderate involvement requires amniocentesis every 1–2 weeks with delivery when fetal lung maturity can be demonstrated (*see* Chap. 7). Severe disease requires weekly amniocentesis and may also require intrauterine transfusion. In all cases assessment of fetal well-being is necessary (*see* Chap. 17).

Ultrasonography

With advances in fetal ultrasonography, assessment of blood flow in the middle cerebral artery now allows for noninvasive assessment of fetal status. The decrease in blood viscosity (due to red blood cell lysis) results in higher velocity blood flow. Normalized values correlated with fetal hematocrit allow for identification affected fetuses with moderate or severe anemia.

Percutaneous Umbilical Blood Sampling

Under circumstances requiring direct measurement of fetal hematocrit, sampling of the umbilical vein allows for such measurement. Normal fetal hematocrit is approximately 40% (36–44%) but may be <30% in severe anemia.

Chapter 14
Infection in Pregnancy

Contents

Background..	114
Symptoms of Infection in Pregnancy...................................	115
Maternal Infection...	115
Fetal Infection...	116
Antibiotic Use in Pregnancy...	117
Sulfonamides..	117
Fluoroquinolones..	118
Aminoglycosides...	118
Vaginitis/Vaginosis...	118
Background..	118
History..	119
Physical Examination..	119
Laboratory Studies..	119
pH *Testing*...	120
KOH *Whiff*..	120
Microscopic Examination..	120
Treatment...	120
Bacterial Vaginosis...	120
Trichomoniasis..	121
Yeast Vaginitis...	121
Gonorrhea/Chlamydia...	121
Urinary Tract Infections..	122
Background..	122
Diagnosis...	122
History...	122
Physical Examination..	123
Laboratory Examination..	123
Treatment...	123
Group B Strep...	124
Background..	124
Diagnosis...	124
Universal Screening...	125
Treatment...	125

© Springer Nature Switzerland AG 2020
P. Lyons, N. McLaughlin, *Obstetrics in Family Medicine*, Current Clinical Practice,
https://doi.org/10.1007/978-3-030-39888-0_14

Key Points
1. Infectious complications in pregnancy include maternal or fetal morbidity, teratogenic or developmental abnormalities, and disruption of the course of pregnancy.
2. Management of infection during pregnancy begins with thorough preconception evaluation.
3. Routine screening of all prenatal patients for common asymptomatic infections is a cornerstone of prenatal care.
4. Women should be screened by history for signs or symptoms that are suggestive of common infectious complications of pregnancy at each prenatal visit.

Background

Infection presents a particular challenge in pregnancy. Symptoms of infection may be subtle, unusual in presentation, or masked by other pregnancy-related symptoms. Infection may affect both the mother and fetus; antibiotic choices may be limited by concerns related to pregnancy and fetal development. As with most elements of obstetrical care, management of infection in pregnancy ideally begins in the preconception period. The preconception history can provide important data concerning infection risk such as recent exposures (toxoplasmosis, tuberculosis, cytomegalovirus), immunization status (influenza, measles, and varicella), and chronic infectious conditions (HIV, herpes, viral hepatitis). For some of these infections, appropriate preconception planning and risk reduction are the only effective intervention. A thorough physical examination may reveal evidence of such infections as active herpes, gonorrhea, or chlamydia. Preconception screening for HIV, tuberculosis, and syphilis, among other conditions, may allow for treatment prior to pregnancy, thereby decreasing the likelihood of adverse prenatal outcomes.

Infections occurring during the course of pregnancy may have two significant consequences. Direct maternal–fetal transmission may lead to infection not just in the mother but also in the fetus. Such infections may have very serious consequences for the fetus or newborn. Herpetic infection in newborns, for example, is associated with a 50% mortality rate and significant morbidity among those infants who survive. In addition, some infectious agents are known to cause complications in the course of pregnancy, particularly preterm labor. Although most studies have shown conflicting data concerning the demonstrated benefit of diagnosis and treatment, most authorities recommend screening and treatment.

Symptoms of Infection in Pregnancy

Although diagnosis of infection in pregnancy is critically important, symptoms of infection in prenatal patients may be absent or difficult to detect or interpret. Many infectious etiologies are asymptomatic. Syphilis, latent-phase herpes, HIV, and others may be present without producing any symptoms in the pregnant patient. For these conditions, routine screening is recommended for all pregnant patients by history, physical examination, and/or diagnostic studies.

Some disease processes produce characteristic symptoms, which should be further evaluated whenever present. Such symptoms as fever, chills, bleeding per vagina, severe abdominal pain, or dysuria should lead to prompt evaluation. For other disease processes, the symptoms associated with infection may be difficult to interpret or may be masked by some of the common symptoms associated with pregnancy. Cervical mucus production may be increased during pregnancy, and some women may interpret this increased mucus as infectious in cause. By contrast, some women may interpret an abnormal vaginal discharge as "normal" for pregnancy, delaying evaluation or failing to mention such symptoms during the course of prenatal care. Nonspecific abdominal pain is also a relatively common symptom occurring during pregnancy. Providers should be diligent in eliciting suggestive symptoms and should maintain a low threshold for following up such symptoms with appropriate diagnostic tests. As a general rule, women should be screened by history for symptoms that are suggestive of common infectious complications of pregnancy at each prenatal visit. Those patients who report such symptoms should be further evaluated for the possible presence of infection (Table 14.1).

Maternal Infection

The primary concern in pregnancy is the health and welfare of the mother. Timely diagnosis and treatment of infection has direct health consequences for the mother and should be approached in the same manner as in nonpregnant patients. Routine prenatal care includes screening for gonorrhea, chlamydia, syphilis, HIV, hepatitis B, and urine culture for bacteriuria. These tests are performed in all patients regardless of symptoms. It is worth noting that most of these infections are sexually transmitted. Pregnancy can be taken as good evidence of unprotected sexual activity and therefore confers the infection risk associated with unprotected sex. Prenatal patients are also routinely screened for evidence of human papilloma virus through Pap smear screening. Although treatment is generally deferred until the patient is no longer pregnant, documentation of the presence and severity of dysplastic lesions is an important element of the comprehensive care plan. The timing and method of screening for these infectious conditions are reviewed in Chap. 3.

Table 14.1 Antibiotics in pregnancy

Infection	Antibiotics
Gram positive	Penicillins
	First-generation cephalosporins
	Clindamycin
Gram negative	Aminoglycosides (*see* text)
	Third-generation cephalosporins
Anaerobic	Clindamycin
Special conditions	
Urinary tract infection	Cephalosporins
	Nitrofurantoin
	Ampicillin (*see* text)
	Sulfisoxazole (*see* text)
Chlamydia	Erythromycin
	Azithromycin
Gonorrhea	Ceftriaxone
Syphilis	Penicillin
Yeast	Azole antifungal agents after the first trimester
Bacterial vaginosis	Clindamycin
	Metronidazole after the first trimester
Trichomoniasis	Metronidazole after the first trimester
Herpes	Acyclovir; cesarean section indicated if present at time of labor
HIV	*See* Chap. 16
Group B strep	Ampicillin in labor

Patients with suggestive symptoms may also be screened for other infectious conditions. Patients with vaginal discharge should be evaluated for the presence of bacterial vaginosis and trichomoniasis in addition to gonorrhea and chlamydia. The presence of bacterial vaginosis has been associated with an increased risk of preterm contractions and preterm labor. Treatment of bacterial vaginosis or trichomoniasis is recommended after the first trimester. Patients with urinary symptoms such as dysuria or hematuria should be evaluated for possible urinary tract infection (UTI).

Fetal Infection

In addition to maternal considerations, many infectious processes have health consequences for the developing fetus. Infection in pregnancy may result in three related fetal complications: direct infection of the fetus or newborn, alteration in the normal course of pregnancy, and alteration of fetal development. Many maternal infections can be transmitted to the fetus either during pregnancy or at the time of delivery. Syphilis, gonorrhea, group B strep (GBS), and HIV, among others, all have demonstrated maternal–fetal transmission. Syphilis is associated with neonatal long bone infection; gonorrhea may cause neonatal ophthalmological disease; GBS is a significant contributor to neonatal febrile illness including meningitis; maternal–fetal transmission of HIV remains a critical source of new HIV infections in many parts of the world.

Infectious agents may result in pregnancy complications even in the absence of direct fetal infection. Maternal infections, such as bacterial vaginosis or GBS, may affect the course of pregnancy resulting in such complications as preterm labor and delivery. Universal or directed screening of prenatal patients can identify a significant number of patients at risk. Several infectious complications have been associated with significant developmental abnormalities in fetuses. Cytomegalovirus, toxoplasmosis, and measles all have potentially serious effects on fetal development. Appropriate screening for exposure and/or timely vaccination can reduce the risk for these complications.

Antibiotic Use in Pregnancy

Antibiotic choice in pregnancy is complicated by the fact that several commonly used classes of antibiotics are contraindicated or should be used with caution in pregnancy. Prior to the use of any antibiotic in pregnancy, providers should review its safety and efficacy in pregnancy. If questions concerning safety remain, consultation with a maternal–fetal expert is recommended. A more complete review of the use of medications in pregnancy can be found in Chap. 4.

Although microbial sensitivity to antibiotics is important in the management of any patient, it is of particular importance in pregnant patients. The potentially limited number of available choices makes culture and sensitivity studies critical in pregnancy. Allergies to such common antibiotics as penicillin may further limit antibiotic choices. In such circumstances, providers may be considering third- or fourth-line antibiotic choices. Under such circumstances, knowing the specific microbe and its sensitivity to available antibiotics is often very helpful.

Although a comprehensive review of all antibiotic classes is beyond the scope of this text, a few key classes should be reviewed (a review of the risk classification for drugs used in pregnancy can be found in Chap. 4).

Sulfonamides

Sulfonamides are most commonly used as sulfamethoxazole in combination with trimethoprim. This antibiotic is routinely used for respiratory tract and UTIs in nonpregnant patients. Sulfonamides readily cross the placenta, and levels persist in newborns for several days postpartum. Sulfonamides are a category B drug early in pregnancy but are category D near term. Complications include jaundice and hemolytic anemia.

Currently available data do not suggest teratogenesis with the use of sulfonamides. Trimethoprim also crosses the placenta freely. Trimethoprim acts as a folate antagonist and may theoretically contribute to congenital abnormalities if used in the first trimester. There is no definitive data linking trimethoprim to congenital defect; however, because of its mechanism of action and some data to suggest a possible increased risk, trimethoprim is a category C drug.

Fluoroquinolones

This class of drugs includes such agents as ciprofloxacin, levofloxacin, lomefloxacin, norfloxacin, and ofloxacin. These are used for a wide variety of infections, including UTIs and respiratory tract infections. Ciprofloxacin has been associated with cartilaginous defects in some animal studies. Data from human studies does not demonstrate a consistent pattern of congenital abnormalities. In general, safer alternatives to fluoroquinolones exist for most conditions. Fluoroquinolones are generally a category C drug.

Aminoglycosides

This class of drugs includes such agents as gentamicin, used widely for serious Gram-negative infections. Although aminoglycosides are used when indicated in pregnancy, there are several issues that should be considered prior to their use. Aminoglycosides cross the placenta and are present at significant but reduced levels (compared with maternal serum levels). Gentamicin is associated with nephrotoxicity in laboratory animals, although only one possible case of possible prenatal gentamicin-associated renal disease has been reported in the literature. Ototoxicity has also been reported with gentamicin use, although no cases associated with in utero exposure have been reported. Aminoglycosides are generally considered class C drugs in pregnancy.

Vaginitis/Vaginosis

Background

A number of infectious agents may result in significant discharge per vagina during pregnancy. Many of the etiologic agents have significance in pregnancy; therefore, a search for the cause and appropriate treatment is particularly important in pregnant patients. In the presence of a significant host inflammatory response, this condition is referred to as vaginitis. In other circumstances, the presence of discharge in the absence of inflammation is referred to as vaginosis. Alteration in the normal vaginal environment including change in pH or elimination of normal flora with the use of some antibiotics allows for proliferation of such abnormal flora as *Gardnerella*, *Trichomonas*, or *Candida* species.

Bacterial vaginosis has been associated with a variety of complications in pregnancy including amniotic fluid infection, chorioamnionitis, postpartum endometritis, premature rupture of membranes (rupture of membranes prior to the onset of labor), preterm labor, preterm delivery, and low birth weight. Complications associated with yeast vaginitis are less clearly defined. In addition to the complications just noted, infection with gonorrhea or chlamydia has been associated with maternal–fetal transmission at the time of delivery.

History

A careful history will often assist in elucidation of the underlying cause for symptoms of vaginitis. The most common, and often most prominent, symptom is discharge per vagina. Patients should also be questioned concerning systemic symptoms such as fever, nausea, vomiting, change in bowel habits, or urinary symptoms. Recent sexual contact should be reviewed (in addition to prior laboratory studies for gonorrhea, chlamydia, urinalysis, urine culture, or wet mount studies). Symptoms in the partner should also be elicited. A review of recent medications and a past history of similar complaints may yield additional information.

Physical Examination

In addition to the routine elements of a prenatal physical examination, a focused exam should be performed to identify key findings consistent with vaginitis or, less commonly, significant peritoneal infections. On abdominal examination, providers should note pain rebound or guarding. On the pelvic examination, a note should be made of external or internal erythema or edema, discharge (including the quality and quantity of such discharge), blood, vaginal or cervical lesions, cervical motion tenderness, and adnexal masses or tenderness.

Laboratory Studies

Further testing is warranted when discharge is noted on exam. Patients should be screened for gonorrhea and chlamydia, especially in the presence of significant mucopurulent discharge. In addition, a sample of discharge should be obtained and tested for pH, KOH (potassium hydroxide) "whiff", test and microscopic examination with saline and KOH solutions.

pH Testing

pH paper placed directly in discharge may be useful in screening for abnormalities. A pH greater than 4.5 is consistent with bacterial vaginosis or trichomoniasis. A pH less than 4.5 is consistent with yeast.

KOH Whiff

KOH mixed with a sample of the discharge can be helpful in diagnosing bacterial vaginosis. A positive "whiff" test reveals a foul or fishy odor when the KOH is added.

Microscopic Examination

One slide prepared with saline and discharge; one slide prepared with KOH and discharge. The saline-prepared slide may show evidence of bacterial vaginosis (clue cells) or trichomoniasis (flagellated protozoa). KOH will lyse most cellular elements within the discharge, leaving only yeast on the slide. The presence of fungal elements on a KOH-prepared slide is evidence of candidal infection.

Treatment

When an infectious agent is identified, most authorities recommend treatment. The benefits of treatment may include reduction of pregnancy-related complications and/or symptomatic relief for the patient. Care should be exercised to select agents with a good safety profile and proven efficacy in pregnancy. If appropriate treatment is unclear, consultation with a maternal–fetal expert is recommended.

Bacterial Vaginosis

Patients with bacterial vaginosis present with mild or no pruritus, minimal pain, thin gray discharge, pH greater than 4.5, positive whiff test, and clue cells on microscopic examination. Bacterial vaginosis may be treated with clindamycin 2% cream or oral clindamycin 300 mg by mouth twice a day for 7 days. After the first trimester, metronidazole is an alternative (0.75% gel 5 g daily for 5 days or 250 mg by mouth three times daily or 500 mg by mouth twice daily for 7 days).

Trichomoniasis

Trichomoniasis presents as mild pruritus, minimal pain, copious yellow thin discharge, pH greater than 4.5, negative whiff test, and flagellated protozoa on microscopic examination. It may be treated after the first trimester with oral metronidazole. Some experts recommend against treating asymptomatic trichomoniasis in pregnancy as studies do not demonstrate improved outcomes. Topical metronidazole is associated with a higher rate of treatment failure and/or recurrence. Treatment is 500 mg of oral metronidazole twice a day for 7 days. An alternative regimen is 2 g of oral metronidazole as a single dose. This regimen is associated with a higher recurrence rate and increased gastrointestinal side effects. Tinidazole is effective in nonpregnant patients, but safety data in pregnancy is limited, and therefore it is not currently recommended.

Yeast Vaginitis

Patients with yeast vaginitis present with mild–severe pruritus, perineal irritation or pain, thick "curd-like" whitish discharge, pH less than 4.5, negative whiff test, and fungal elements on KOH-prepared microscopic examination. Yeast vaginitis may be treated with topical vaginal antifungal preparations, many of which are now available over the counter (OTC). Because of the desirability of obtaining a clear diagnosis and of minimizing the use of unnecessary medications during pregnancy, most patients should be cautioned against self-treating with OTC preparations without consulting their provider.

Gonorrhea/Chlamydia

Gonorrhea/chlamydia should be treated in the usual manner to prevent maternal and/or fetal complications. In pregnancy, the use of quinolones and most variants of tetracyclines should be avoided. Gonorrhea should be treated with dual therapy including ceftriaxone and azithromycin. In the case of cephalosporin allergy, recommendations include either (1) desensitization followed by treatment with cephalosporin or (2) azithromycin 2 g orally. This treatment is also effective for chlamydia but has lower efficacy against gonorrhea and therefore should be followed by a test of cure. Treatment for chlamydia is either azithromycin 1 g orally as a single dose or amoxicillin 500 mg orally three times daily for 7 days. Because treatment efficacy is reduced in pregnancy, a test of cure is recommended no sooner than 3 weeks following treatment.

Urinary Tract Infections

Background

Infections of both the lower and upper urinary tracts are more common in pregnancy. Anatomic and hormonal changes associated with pregnancy increase urinary stasis and may enhance ascending bacterial seeding. The increase in size of the uterus combined, later in pregnancy, with the presence of fetal body parts yields a functional partial obstruction of the outflow tract thereby increasing urinary stasis. Increased progesterone may yield ureteral smooth muscle relaxation, thus increasing the risk for ascending bacterial seeding and proliferation. Such changes appear to peak late in the second trimester or early in the third trimester. UTIs are associated with an increased risk of preterm delivery and low birth weight. In addition, the bacterial seeding can have serious consequences for the mother, including cystitis and pyelonephritis.

Women often report increased urinary frequency during the course of pregnancy. However, bacteriuria and its sequelae are also common during pregnancy. Approximately 5–10% of all pregnant women develop asymptomatic bacteriuria (with higher prevalence among some at-risk populations). Of these, approximately one-third will develop clinically significant UTIs if not treated. Cystitis complicates about 1% of all pregnancies with an additional 1–2% of all pregnant women developing pyelonephritis. Commonly occurring pathogens include *E. coli* (80%), *Klebsiella*, *Proteus*, and *Staphylococcus saprophyticus*. GBS is an uncommon cause of UTIs but is of particular significance in pregnancy because of its association with an increased risk for preterm labor and neonatal infection.

Diagnosis

The challenge, then, in pregnancy is to distinguish "normal" pregnancy-related urinary frequency from the urinary symptoms (including frequency) associated with UTIs.

Asymptomatic bacteriuria, mentioned above, does necessitate treatment to prevent complications that can result from infection. This is diagnosed with a screening urine culture, ideally in the first trimester of pregnancy. Office urine point of care dip and formal urinalysis should not be used for this screening as they lack the sensitivity and specificity for diagnosis in an asymptomatic population. Culture results should be used to guide antibiotic treatment for results with $\leq 10^5$ bacterial cfu/ml. Treatment duration should be 3–7 days.

History

Many patients may be asymptomatic. Others may report urinary frequency and urgency; dysuria; hematuria; fever; abdominal pain, cramping, or contractions; and flank or back pain. Although frequency and urgency may be normal in pregnancy, the presence of the other symptoms should always prompt further evaluation. A change in baseline frequency or urgency should also prompt reevaluation. Because of the subtle or potentially confusing nature of the patients' presenting complaints, providers should maintain a high index of suspicion for UTI. The presence of any symptoms should generally prompt evaluation and treatment if indicated.

Physical Examination

The physical examination should focus on physical signs of infection and/or signs of ascending infection. Key elements of the physical examination should include temperature, abdominal pain, rebound or guarding, and costovertebral angle tenderness. A pelvic examination is indicated for patients who present with abdominal or back symptoms or for those who report bleeding, contractions, or cramping.

Laboratory Examination

Urine culture remains the gold standard for diagnosis of UTIs. More than 100,000 colony-forming units per milliliter are considered a positive urine culture. In addition to assisting with the diagnosis, culture may also be useful in identifying the bacterial etiology and the antibiotic sensitivities of the isolated organism. More rapid assessment is often necessary, however, and a variety of additional tests are available that can provide results while the patient is still in the office (or within a few hours). Collection of a clean catch specimen can be difficult for the patient; nevertheless it is important, as collection can significantly alter the diagnostic utility of the test and thus treatment plans. Formal urinalysis performed in a laboratory may be helpful in assisting in diagnosis.

Other office-based tests are very specific but not sensitive. Dipstick leukocyte esterase testing is approximately 20% sensitive and 95% specific. Dipstick nitrite is approximately 57% sensitive and 95% specific. Urine microscopy with more than ten white blood cells per high-power field on a spun urine sample is about 25% sensitive and 99% specific. These tests can be very useful if positive but may need to be followed up with urine culture if negative.

Treatment

Because of the potentially significant complications of untreated UTIs, treatment is recommended regardless of patient symptoms. There are several treatment options, but, as always, each treatment option should be reviewed for safety and efficacy in pregnancy. Ampicillin has traditionally been the treatment of choice for UTIs during pregnancy. Its safety profile is excellent, and it has been used widely during pregnancy. However, emerging ampicillin resistance in *E. coli* (more than one-third resistant in some regions) has led many providers to use alternatives as first-line therapy. Among the options for treatment are the following:

- Cephalexin (category B, 250–500 mg orally, twice a day)
- Nitrofurantoin (category B except contraindicated in term pregnancies), 50–100 mg orally, twice a day)
- Sulfa drugs (sulfisoxazole 1 g orally, four times a day; TMP/SMZ 160/180 mg orally, twice a day; they may be used in the second trimester but should be avoided in either first or third trimester)
- Fosfomycin (category B; 3 g single dose)

With the exception of fosfomycin, all treatment should be for 3–7 days for lower tract infections and up to 2 weeks for pyelonephritis.

Group B Strep

Background

GBS (most commonly *Streptococcus agalactiae*) are normal colonic flora. Under appropriate conditions, GBS colonize in the vagina, complicating pregnancy and the early neonatal course. Of all pregnant women, 10–30% are colonized with GBS in either the vaginal or rectal areas. GBS is a common and significant cause of prenatal and neonatal morbidity. GBS is associated with preterm labor, premature rupture of membranes, and preterm delivery. Less commonly, GBS is associated with UTIs. It is also associated with neonatal infection, including meningitis. Infants born to colonized women often develop early-onset invasive disease, 80% within the first 7 days of life. The prevalence of invasive disease is about 0.6 per 1000 live births. In the United States, GBS is responsible for about 2000 neonatal infections and 100 fatalities annually.

Treatment of GBS has been shown to decrease the incidence of such complications. The use of intrapartum antibiotic therapy to treat women at increased risk for transmission to their newborns can significantly reduce peripartum transmission and neonatal infection. Treatment of invasive GBS infection is associated with a reduction in rates of premature rupture of membranes and preterm delivery. The key to successful management is identification and treatment of those patients who are at risk for preterm complications or peripartum transmission.

Diagnosis

Diagnosis of GBS can be challenging. Most patients do not consistently demonstrate colonization throughout the course of pregnancy. Early GBS cultures do not correlate well with GBS status at the time of delivery. In addition, patients colonized with GBS are generally asymptomatic. For this reason, authorities recommend universal screening of prenatal patients regardless of risk or symptoms near term (36 + 0 to 37+ 6 weeks' gestation). For patients who present with suggestive signs or symptoms, GBS testing should be performed. High-risk conditions include pre-term labor, premature rupture of membranes, or evidence of GBS UTI. Those patients with a past history of premature rupture of membranes, preterm delivery, or neonatal strep infection should also be considered high risk.

Universal Screening

All patients are screened during the course of pregnancy with treatment reserved for those who have positive cultures or who are at high risk.

- GBS testing is performed on all women at 36 weeks–37 weeks' + 6 days gesta-tion (the results of which more nearly correlate with intrapartum GBS status than cultures obtained earlier in pregnancy).
- In the absence of GBS culture results, all patients with fever, prolonged rupture of membranes (>18 h), or gestational age less than 37 weeks should be presumed GBS positive.
- In the absence of GBS cultures, all patients with a past history of GBS UTI or neonatal GBS infection should be presumed GBS positive.
- In patients with preterm premature rupture of membranes, GBS cultures should be obtained. Patients may be presumed GBS positive until culture results are available.

Treatment

Penicillin is the gold standard treatment for GBS in patients without penicillin allergy. Acceptable penicillin-based regimens include penicillin G intravenous, 5 million units loading dose followed by 2.5 million intravenous units every 4 h until delivery or 2 g of ampicillin intravenous loading dose followed by 1 g intravenously every 4 h.

For patients with a non-serious penicillin sensitivity, cefazolin 2 g IV once and then 1 g IV every 8 h until delivery is recommended. Alternatives for patients with more significant penicillin allergies include clindamycin (if sensitivity data is avail-able and indicates clindamycin sensitivity) or vancomycin 20 mg/kg every 12 h (max 2 g dose). A useful and increasingly available tool for determining allergy severity is the penicillin allergy skin test. This is safe in pregnancy and can be espe-cially useful in patients who have an unknown allergy severity.

Chapter 15
Hypertension in Pregnancy

Contents

Background.. 128
Diagnosis... 128
   Diagnostic Criteria.. 128
   History.. 130
   Physical Examination... 130
   Laboratory Studies.. 130
Management... 131
   Chronic Hypertension... 131
Pre-eclampsia... 131
   Prevention... 131
   Management.. 131
   Seizure Prevention... 133
   Postpartum Management... 134

Key Points

1. Hypertension in pregnancy is defined as blood pressure (BP) higher than 140 mmHg systolic or 90 mmHg diastolic on two occasions separated by at least 6 h.
2. Pregnancy-induced hypertension is defined as hypertension diagnosed at or after 20 weeks' gestation.
3. Pre-eclampsia is a multisystem disease characterized by hypertension and proteinuria.
4. Pre-eclampsia may lead to fetal complications including preterm delivery, intrauterine growth restriction (IUGR), fetal demise, and perinatal death, as well as maternal complications of seizure, stroke, and death.

© Springer Nature Switzerland AG 2020

P. Lyons, N. McLaughlin, *Obstetrics in Family Medicine*, Current Clinical Practice,
https://doi.org/10.1007/978-3-030-39888-0_15

Background

Pregnancy may be complicated by hypertension either as a pre-existing condition or as a newly diagnosed condition during pregnancy. Each condition carries with it significant risks and important management considerations that may impact the well-being of both the mother and fetus. Pre-eclampsia, a multisystem disorder that is marked by pregnancy-induced hypertension and evidence of end organ involvement, is a significant obstetrical risk that affects approximately 5% of pregnancies. Evidence of end organ involvement may include proteinuria, thrombocytopenia, visual complaints, pulmonary edema, or impaired hepatic function. Proteinuria has traditionally been considered the hallmark of pre-eclampsia but is not necessary for the diagnosis.

The exact cause of pre-eclampsia is unknown, but its multisystem complications are well described. Physiologically, pre-eclampsia is marked by increased vascular resistance, platelet aggregation, and endothelial dysfunction. Clinically, pre-eclampsia may be identified with hypertension (occurring after 20 weeks' gestation), proteinuria, HELLP syndrome (*h*emolysis, *e*levated *l*iver enzymes, *l*ow *p*latelets), and seizures (eclampsia).

Chronic hypertension is defined as hypertension (repeated BP readings of systolic ≥ 140 or diastolic ≥ 90 mmHg) existing prior to pregnancy or first diagnosed prior to 20 weeks' gestation. Obstetrical complications associated with chronic hypertension include increased risk for pre-eclampsia (discussed later), abruptio placentae, premature delivery, IUGR, fetal demise, and fetal stress. Pregnancy itself may worsen hypertensive renal disease. The majority of such complications occur in women with diastolic BPs higher than 110 mmHg although such complications may occur in women with lower BP.

Pre-eclampsia occurs in approximately 5% of all pregnancies and may be associated with many of the same obstetrical risks as chronic hypertension (Table 15.1): HELLP syndrome (10–20%), abruptio placentae (1–4%), and eclampsia (<1%). Rarely, it may also be associated with maternal stroke or death. Complications for the neonate include IUGR (10–25%), preterm delivery (15–67%), and perinatal death (1–2%). For both the mother and infant, the presence of pre-eclampsia may be associated with long-term cardiovascular morbidity.

Diagnosis

Diagnostic Criteria

The diagnostic criteria for hypertension in pregnant patients are similar to those for nonpregnant patients. Hypertension may be diagnosed in patients with at least two BP readings of more than 140 mmHg systolic or more than 90 mmHg diastolic separated by at least 4 h but not more than 7 days.

Table 15.1 Risk factors for pre-eclampsia

Maternal
Family history of pre-eclampsia
Early or late maternal age
Nulliparity
Prior history of pre-eclampsia
Assisted reproduction
Vascular disease
Diabetes
Obesity
Hypertension
Renal disease
Thrombophilia
Rheumatic disease
Infection
Paternal
Primipaternity
Prior pregnancy complicated by pre-eclampsia
Donated sperm
Fetal
Multifetal gestation
Hydrops fetalis
Chromosomal abnormalities
Congenital abnormalities

Pre-eclampsia is diagnosed by a combination of hypertension first diagnosed after 20 weeks' gestation and proteinuria ($\geq$300 mg per 24 h or 1+ dipstick protein in two random urine samples separated by at least 4 h). Diagnosis of pre-eclampsia can be made in the absence of proteinuria if severe criteria are present. Hypertension with systolic >160 or diastolic >110 is considered diagnostic. In addition, hypertension associated with neurological (headache, visual changes, altered mental status), hepatic dysfunction including elevated liver enzymes (>2 times upper limit of normal transaminase), renal dysfunction (creatinine >1.1 mg.dL or 2 times baseline), pulmonary edema, or hematological (decreased platelet count) findings is also diagnostic. Ten percent of patients who develop HELLP syndrome and up to 33% of patients who develop eclampsia will not demonstrate the traditional findings of both hypertension and proteinuria.

Severe pre-eclampsia is diagnosed if any one of the three criteria (hypertension, proteinuria, multiorgan involvement) is severe. The criterion for severe hypertension in pregnancy is a systolic BP >160 mmHg and/or diastolic BP >110 mmHg. Proteinuria is considered severe at levels 5 g or more per day. Multiorgan involvement may be demonstrated by pulmonary edema, seizures, altered mental status, headaches, visual disturbance, persistent right upper quadrant pain with elevated liver enzymes, oliguria (<500 cc/day), or thrombocytopenia (<100,000).

History

Although the diagnosis of pre-eclampsia is generally made on the basis of BP readings and proteinuria, a number of risk factors have been identified and should be reviewed in the history. These risk factors are shown in Table 15.2 and include family history of pre-eclampsia, past history of pre-eclampsia, nulliparity, primi-paternity, age over 40, assisted fertility, multiple gestation, chronic hypertension, diabetes mellitus, renal disease, thrombophilia obesity, maternal infection, and smoking.

In addition, all patients should be screened at each visit for symptoms suggestive of possible pre-eclampsia including headache, visual changes, altered mental status, abdominal pain, nausea, or vomiting.

Physical Examination

Each prenatal visit should include documentation of the patient's BP. For patients who demonstrate elevated BP, a return visit should be scheduled within 1 week for a recheck of BP.

For patients with elevated BP, the physical examination should also include ophthalmological, neurological, and abdominal examinations as well as notation of peripheral edema (feet, hands, and face).

Laboratory Studies

The most accurate test for proteinuria is a 24-h urine collection with measurement of protein excretion. In settings where such collections are not practical, two separate dipstick urinalysis tests demonstrating at least 1+ protein may substitute. Additional labs for patients with suspected pre-eclampsia should include complete blood count with platelets, liver enzymes, and a coagulation panel.

Table 15.2 Complications of pre-eclampsia	
	Preterm delivery
	Intrauterine growth restriction
	HELLP syndrome
	Pulmonary edema
	Acute renal failure
	Abruptio placentae
	Perinatal death
	Eclampsia
	Stroke
	Death

Management

Chronic Hypertension

Patients with a pre-existing diagnosis of hypertension should continue to receive treatment during the course of pregnancy. Providers should review the safety of their existing antihypertensive regimen and make adjustments as necessary. Antihypertensive medications are reviewed in Chap. 4. Antihypertensive medications commonly used during pregnancy include methyldopa, nifedipine, and β-blockers. For patients diagnosed with hypertension after conception but prior to 20 weeks' gestation, the role of antihypertensives is less clear. Patients with severe hypertension (diastolic over 110 mmHg) should receive pharmacological treatment, but treatment of women with mild essential hypertension in pregnancy has not been shown to improve outcomes. Intravenous labetalol or hydralazine and oral nifedipine are appropriate options for management of severe hypertension in pregnancy. Patients with chronic hypertension should be carefully followed for signs or symptoms of pre-eclampsia as 15–25% will develop superimposed pre-eclampsia.

Pre-eclampsia

Prevention

As the risk factors associated with increased risk for pre-eclampsia have become increasingly well defined, interest has been focused on prevention of pre-eclampsia in patients at high risk. Proposed interventions have included dietary supplements, aspirin, and antihypertensive medications. Although the results have been mixed, there is little evidence to support the preventive benefits of diet and exercise, protein or salt restriction, magnesium, fish oil or antioxidant supplementation, heparin, or antihypertensive medications. Low-dose aspirin has been shown to provide small to moderate benefit. The benefit appears to be risk dependent (greatest benefit is noted among patients at highest risk). Calcium supplementation has been shown to provide benefit in populations at risk for low dietary calcium. The benefit in developed countries, including the United States, is not clear.

Management

The management of pre-eclampsia involves balancing the maternal risks of prolonged pregnancy against the neonatal risks of premature delivery. The potential risks and benefits for each patient must be considered individually. Although no universally acceptable management protocol can be recommended, a general approach to the management of pre-eclampsia is outlined in Fig. 15.1.

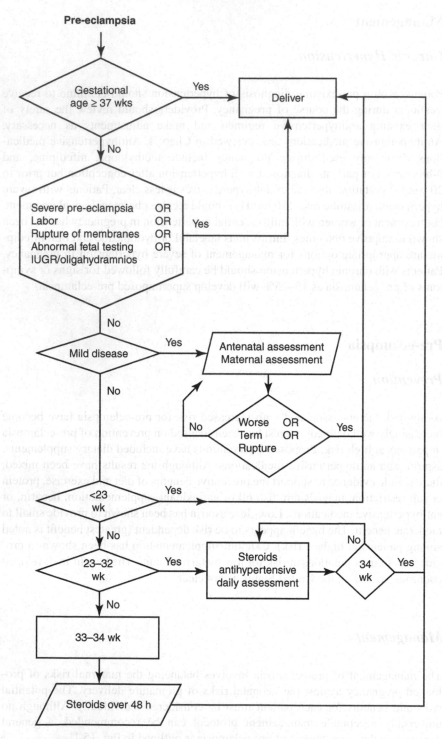

Fig. 15.1 Management of pre-eclampsia

Delivery is the definitive maternal management plan. For this reason, delivery should occur as soon as it can reasonably be achieved. For patients at term with mild disease, induction of labor is indicated. For patients with severe pre-eclampsia at or beyond 34 weeks, delivery is indicated with appropriate neonatal support. If the maternal condition appears stable but there is evidence of fetal compromise, management should follow a protocol similar to that of IUGR (*see* Chap. 6).

For patients with mild disease, no evidence of fetal compromise, and a gestational age of less than 34 weeks, ideal management is not well established. Under these circumstances, careful monitoring of maternal condition should be combined with close evaluation of fetal well-being. If both maternal and fetal conditions remain stable, delivery can occur at 37 weeks. If either maternal or fetal condition worsens, delivery should occur as soon as possible.

As noted for chronic hypertension, the use of antihypertensives has shown mixed results. For patients with severe hypertension, the use of antihypertensive medications has been shown to reduce maternal complications. However, such treatment has not been shown to reduce neonatal complications and does not alter the maternal course of disease in relation to multiorgan complications. The use of antihypertensives has not been shown to improve maternal or neonatal outcomes in patients with mild disease. There is little evidence to support the use of any specific class of antihypertensive medications in the treatment of pre-eclampsia. Several medications are contraindicated in pregnancy however. These include angiotensin converting enzyme inhibitors (ACE) and angiotensin II receptor blockers due to associated IUGR, oligohydramnios, and death as well as atenolol due to associated IUGR. Thiazide diuretics are generally not started during pregnancy but may be continued during pregnancy. If used during pregnancy, thiazide diuretics should be discontinued if the patient develops preeclampsia.

The use of corticosteroids has not been shown to improve maternal outcomes, although their use has been shown to improve neonatal outcomes for infants born prior to 34 weeks' gestation.

Seizure Prevention

Seizure (eclampsia) is one of the most significant complications of pre-eclampsia and may occur without preceding warning signs. For this reason, seizure prophylaxis with magnesium sulfate is indicated for patients with pre-eclampsia in the intrapartum period. Specific regimens for the use of magnesium may vary between institutions, and the specific protocol should be reviewed by each provider. One possible protocol is as follows: loading dose of 6 g of intravenous magnesium sulfate followed by 2 g per hour of continuous intravenous infusion. Magnesium may be toxic in high doses, and patients should be monitored closely while undergoing magnesium therapy. Maternal BP, deep tendon reflexes, mental status, and urinary output should be monitored. Serum magnesium levels should be measured. Magnesium levels above 7 mEq/L are associated with diminished deep tendon reflexes. Magnesium levels above 10 mEq/L are associated with respiratory depression.

Magnesium levels above 12 mEq/L are associated with cardiac depression and arrest. Magnesium elevation is reversible with 10% calcium gluconate 10 mL intravenous given over 10–15 min.

Postpartum Management

Although the primary concern in the management of gestational hypertension and pre-eclampsia is during the pregnancy, maternal risk extends beyond delivery. Because the risk of postpartum eclampsia is highest in the first 24–48 hours following delivery, patients managed with MgSO4 should continue treatment for 12–24 hours after delivery. Blood pressure should be closely monitored while the patient remains in the hospital. Most patients will demonstrate significant diuresis, decrease in blood pressure, and relief of symptoms (if any); however patients with persistent blood pressure above 150 mmHg systolic or 100 mmHg diastolic should be carefully monitored. Patients with blood pressure greater than 160 mmHg systolic or 110 mmHg diastolic should receive antihypertensive medication. Following discharge, patients should have blood pressure rechecked within a week.

Chapter 16
Diabetes in Pregnancy

Contents

Background... 135
Diagnosis.. 136
Pregestational Diabetes.. 137
    Management.. 137
Management in Pregnancy.. 138
Diet... 138
Insulin.. 139
Oral Hypoglycemics.. 139
Blood Sugar Monitoring.. 139
Gestational Diabetes.. 140
    Preconception Management.. 140
Management in Pregnancy... 140
Management in Labor... 141
Postpartum Management... 141

Key Points
1. Diabetes mellitus (DM) is defined as carbohydrate intolerance resulting from either insulin deficiency or insulin insensitivity.
2. Exposure to elevated serum glucose is associated with increased risk for organogenic birth defects, macrosomic infants, shoulder dystocia, and birth trauma.
3. Gestational diabetes is defined as glucose intolerance first recognized during pregnancy.

Background

DM (hyperglycemia secondary to either insulin deficiency or relative insulin insensitivity) is a significant medical condition with a potentially profound impact on pregnancy. Uncontrolled diabetes prior to or early in the course of pregnancy is

© Springer Nature Switzerland AG 2020
P. Lyons, N. McLaughlin, *Obstetrics in Family Medicine*, Current Clinical Practice,
https://doi.org/10.1007/978-3-030-39888-0_16

Table 16.1 Congenital
abnormalities associated with
diabetes

Duodenal and anorectal atresia
Hydronephrosis
Renal agenesis
Neural tube defects
Anencephaly
Ventricular septal defects
Aortic coarctation
Transposition of the great vessels

associated with a variety of birth defects, including renal, gastrointestinal, cardiac, central nervous system, and skeletal abnormalities (*see* Table 16.1). The presence of diabetes may alter the interpretation of some prenatal tests including α-fetoprotein and obstetric triple screen. Pregnancy may, in turn, affect the course of diabetes, worsening glucose control in patients with pre-existing diabetes.

DM may be classified as type 1 diabetes, associated with pancreatic failure and insulin deficiency; type 2 diabetes, associated with ineffective insulin utilization (generally associated with hyperinsulinemia); or gestational diabetes mellitus (GDM), which is diabetes first diagnosed or recognized in pregnancy (generally associated with insulin resistance and similar to type 2 diabetes). GDM is associated with increased glucose intolerance during the course of pregnancy. In most cases this glucose intolerance will resolve following pregnancy. Hormonal changes associated with pregnancy increase maternal glucose intolerance. Human placental lactogen decreases cellular glucose uptake and increases lipolysis. Estrogen and progesterone are also known to affect glucose metabolism although to a lesser extent than human placental lactogen.

Diagnosis

Diagnosis of types 1 and 2 DM is made prior to pregnancy. The diagnosis is made on the basis of documented hyperglycemia with either insulin deficiency (type 1) or insulin resistance (type 2). The diagnosis of GDM is generally made on the basis of oral glucose testing during the course of prenatal care, although, in some cases, the diagnosis may be made on the basis of fasting blood glucose values.

Screening for GDM is an area of some controversy. Most authorities including the United States Preventive Services Task Force recommend universal screening of all patients at 24–28 weeks' gestation. Earlier testing for those patients identified as high risk (*see* Table 16.2) is suggested by some authorities but has limited data demonstrating improved outcomes.

Initial screening is via 50 g glucose tolerance testing. Patients are not required to fast and do not need to alter their dietary intake. A standardized 50 g glucose load is administered orally, and serum glucose level is tested at 1 h. The threshold for a positive screening test is also an area of some controversy, and providers should be aware of the standard of care in their institution. Serum glucose values should be less than 130 or 140 mg/dL. The lower value has a higher sensitivity (will miss

Table 16.2 Risk factors for gestational diabetes

| Family history of diabetes |
| Family history of macrosomic infants |
| Ethnicity |
| Obesity |
| Past history of gestational diabetes |
| Past history of macrosomic infant |
| Multigestation |

Table 16.3 Gestational diabetes diagnosis (100 g, 3 h oral glucose tolerance test)

Sample	Threshold
Fasting	95
1 h	180
2 h	155
3 h	140

Note: the diagnosis of gestational diabetes is made if any two values exceed the values listed in the table

fewer true cases of diabetes) but is associated with a higher false-positive rate. The higher value reduces false-positive findings (has a higher specificity) but may have a lower sensitivity.

Regardless of which threshold is used, all patients with a positive screening test should undergo diagnostic testing with a 3 h 100 g oral glucose challenge test. Patients should eat a carbohydrate-rich or unrestricted diet for 3 days prior to testing but should fast the night before the test. A standardized 100 g oral glucose load is administered, and serum glucose levels are drawn fasting 1, 2, and 3 h following administration. There is debate concerning the threshold values for this test as well. The American College of Obstetricians and Gynecologists' recommendation is presented in Table 16.3. According to this protocol, blood glucose levels should be below 95 mg/dL fasting and below 185 mg/dL, 155 mg/dL, and 140 mg/dL at 1 h, 2 h, and 3 h, respectively. The test is considered diagnostic if any two values exceed the threshold.

Pregestational Diabetes

Management

Preconception Management

The management of pregestational diabetes ideally should begin during the preconception period. Preconception management should include discussion of the effects of diabetes on pregnancy as well as discussion of the effects of pregnancy on diabetes. Patients should be counseled concerning the risks of maternal hyperglycemia on the developing infant and the importance of strict glycemic control prior to and throughout the course of pregnancy.

Table 16.4 White's
classification of diabetes in
pregnancy

Class	Definition
A	Diet controlled
B	Age of onset ≥20 years, duration <10 years
C	Age of onset 10–19 years or duration 10–19 years
D	Age of onset <10 or duration >20 years
F	Nephropathy (≥500 mg/day proteinuria)
H	Clinically evident arteriosclerotic heart disease
R	Retinopathy
T	Renal transplant

Preconception management should also include classification of the severity of diabetes. The modified White's classification system is shown in Table 16.4. This classification is based on four factors: (a) treatment regimen, (b) duration of disease or age of onset, (c) associated disease, and (d) diabetic complications.

Because of the association of poor glycemic control with an increased risk for congenital defects, all patients should be intensively monitored and tightly controlled prior to conception. Because of the complexity of achieving tight glycemic control, such efforts should begin well before anticipated conception when possible.

Oral hypoglycemic agents are not generally utilized during pregnancy. Patients managed on oral hypoglycemic agents prior to conception may require additional time (and education) to transition to the use of insulin. Patients may also require comprehensive diabetes education on diet, exercise, and blood glucose self-monitoring. Prenatal vitamins with folate should be prescribed as a part of preconception management as well.

Management in Pregnancy

For patients who did not receive preconception evaluation and treatment, all of the management just discussed should begin with the first prenatal visit. Because the early weeks of pregnancy are the period of organogenesis, rapid assessment and intervention are critical to improve outcomes. Patients may require more frequent visits and will probably benefit from intensive educational interventions, beginning with a review of the patient's own knowledge of her disease and its management.

Diet

All patients with diabetes should be counseled concerning the role of diet in the management of diabetes. Although specific recommendations may vary between patients, general recommendations include the following:

1. Caloric intake per day should be individualized, generally as several small meals rather than fewer large meals.
2. Restriction of simple carbohydrates.
3. Inclusion of complex carbohydrates in an overall diet that includes approximately 40% carbohydrates, 30% fat, and 30% protein.
4. Regular and predictable caloric intake will facilitate glycemic control and reduce the likelihood of hypoglycemia.
5. A small snack should be available at all times in case of hypoglycemia.

Insulin

Pharmacological management of diabetes in pregnancy generally utilizes a combination of intermediate- and short-acting insulin. This combination allows for more controlled adjustment of glycemic control than either oral hypoglycemic agents or long-acting insulin alone. The exact dose of insulin will be based on measured blood glucose values with target levels of less than 105 mg/dL fasting (95 mg/dL according to some authorities) and less than 120 mg/dL 2 h postprandial. Insulin should be adjusted as necessary to achieve these target levels. Tight glycemic control has been demonstrated to improve obstetrical outcomes but has also been associated with increased risk of hypoglycemia. For this reason, patients should be educated concerning the symptoms of hypoglycemia and the appropriate steps to be taken should hypoglycemia occur.

Oral Hypoglycemics

Although insulin has been the traditional pharmacologic treatment choice (and remains the most common choice), there is increasing acceptance of oral hypoglycemic medications in pregnancy. Glyburide and metformin are both considered acceptable for treatment of gestational diabetes when medication is indicated. Data from well-designed studies is limited, but outcomes appear to be similar across each of these medication options.

Blood Sugar Monitoring

As noted, insulin dosing should be based on the results of blood glucose monitoring. For this reason, frequent finger-stick glucose monitoring should be a part of the management of patients treated with insulin. Although glycosylated hemoglobin values may provide adjunctive data concerning the level of glucose control, the long-term (3-month) retrospective nature of such testing makes it unsuitable for insulin management in pregnancy. Patients should be counseled to test blood sugar fasting and 2 h after every meal on a daily basis. Target blood sugar values are <95 mg/dL fasting and <120 mg/dL 2 h postprandial.

If such intense monitoring is not feasible, patients should be counseled to vary daily (e.g., fasting and 2 h after lunch 1 day, 2 h after breakfast and 2 h after dinner the next) to allow for adequate assessment of insulin needs. Additional testing may be recommended at times when patients feel the symptoms of hypoglycemia to document the decrease in glucose levels.

Gestational Diabetes

Preconception Management

Preconception management of GDM begins with assessment of risk factors for the development of diabetes during pregnancy. The risk factors for GDM are listed in Table 16.1. All patients should be screened for risk factors for GDM. Patients found to be at increased risk may benefit from preconceptual diabetes testing as type 2 DM and GDM share common risk factors. Patients discovered to have diabetes prior to becoming pregnant should receive additional preconception counseling as noted earlier.

Management in Pregnancy

Patients with GDM should be managed similarly to those patients with pre-existing diabetes. Although many patients with GDM can be appropriately managed with lifestyle modification alone, all patients should be counseled concerning the indications for further treatment with insulin if necessary. All patients with diabetes should test blood sugar regularly to assess the adequacy of their treatment regimen.

Because of the fetal risks associated with diabetes in pregnancy, all patients with diabetes should begin fetal surveillance in the third trimester of pregnancy. Antenatal assessment is discussed in Chap. 18. In addition, because of the risk of macrosomia, careful assessment of fetal growth should be included in prenatal assessment. Patients with evidence of macrosomic or small-for-gestational-age fetuses should receive ultrasonographic assessment of fetal growth.

Management in Labor

During labor, efforts should be made to maintain the patient's serum glucose levels between 80 and 110 mg/dL. Care should be taken, however, not to induce maternal hypoglycemia in patients who are restricted from eating or drinking during the course of labor. This is especially true for patients with prolonged second-stage labor.

Postpartum Management

All patients diagnosed with GDM should be screened for diabetes 6–12 weeks post-partum. Such patients are at increased risk for subsequent diagnosis of type 2 diabetes and should therefore be screened every 3 years following delivery.

Chapter 17
HIV in Pregnancy

Contents

Preconception Counseling... 144
Initial Pregnancy Evaluation... 144
Antiretroviral Use in Pregnancy... 145
Intrapartum Management.. 146
Postpartum Management.. 147

Key Points
1. All women who are found to be HIV positive during pregnancy should be started on an appropriate antiretroviral regimen as soon as possible.
2. Suppression of the HIV to undetectable levels is the goal prior to conception and throughout the pregnancy.
3. Pregnancy-related physiologic changes may alter the pharmacokinetics of antiretroviral therapy requiring close monitoring of viral load and possible adjustment of dose.
4. HIV infection, regardless of viral load, remains a contraindication to breastfeeding

The management of patients with HIV represents a significant success of modern medicine. A disease that was once nearly universally fatal has now become a disease that is chronically managed. The advent of widespread screening, pre-exposure prophylaxis, and highly active antiretroviral therapy has fundamentally altered medical management landscape for all patients with HIV.

The transition from fatal acute disease to controlled chronic disease has had profound implications for obstetrical management as well. Early studies indicated profound benefit in reducing maternal–fetal transmission with treatment. This has been followed by considerable new knowledge impacting preconception, conception, labor, and postpartum management for women who are pregnant or are considering becoming pregnant.

© Springer Nature Switzerland AG 2020
P. Lyons, N. McLaughlin, *Obstetrics in Family Medicine*, Current Clinical Practice,
https://doi.org/10.1007/978-3-030-39888-0_17

Preconception Counseling

As noted in Chap. 2, preconception care begins nonjudgmental discussions with all women of reproductive age regarding plans, concerns, or questions related to pregnancy. As many pregnancies in the United States are unplanned, this ongoing conversation is best integrated into ongoing primary care. All the routine elements of such preconception dialog pertain to women living with HIV, with the added need to incorporate education and planning for HIV specific concerns.

Issues of concern for women living with HIV and considering pregnancy include disease-related issues, partner-related issues, and infant-related issues. The complexity of these issues may warrant referral to experts in HIV even for providers who routinely care for women living with HIV. For women planning a pregnancy, the following issues should be addressed prior to conception:

Pregnancy health is critically dependent on pre-pregnancy health. In addition to maximizing HIV-related medical management, patients should be counseled on alcohol, tobacco, and drug use (including treatment, if indicated), nutrition (including folate supplementation), and optimizing management of other chronic diseases, if any.

Counseling regarding transmission of HIV both to the infant and potential partners. This includes an understanding of maternal–fetal transmission and reduction of transmission risk during pregnancy, labor, and the postpartum period. It also includes a discussion of risk reduction for transmission with partners (including pre-exposure prophylaxis when appropriate).

Viral suppression to below detectable limits is the goal of therapy prior to conception and throughout the course of the pregnancy. Viral suppression is associated with improved outcomes for both the mother and the infant.

For patients on antiretroviral therapy, a discussion of pregnancy-related concerns with their specific regimen is important. Specifically, risk of neural tube defects associated with dolutegravir should be noted when applicable.

Review of patients for hepatitis B risk including screening if not already performed.

Initial Pregnancy Evaluation

In addition to the routine intake evaluation appropriate for all pregnant patients, women living with HIV will require individualized care based on their specific medical circumstances. Although preconception counseling would best occur prior to presentation for a prenatal evaluation, this is not always the case. For this reason all women living with HIV should review the issues noted above at the first prenatal visit.

In addition, a critical element of the first visit is to review and revise, if needed, the antiretroviral regimen. If not on antiretroviral therapy at the time of presentation, the current recommendation is that all women be started on an appropriate regimen as early in pregnancy as possible. It is also recommended that antiretroviral therapy be continued at all points during the pregnancy including prenatal, peripartum, and postpartum. The goal of therapy, as noted, is viral suppression to undetectable levels.

Antiretroviral drug resistance genotype testing should be used to inform all anti-retroviral therapy selection choices including initiation of therapy and changes in regimen for patients who have not achieved undetectable viral load goals. For pregnant patients not on antiretroviral therapy at the time of pregnancy, the current recommendation is to start antiretroviral therapy prior to obtaining testing. Adjustments may be made to the regimen based on the results of subsequent genotype testing.

Several key pregnancy-related issues should be introduced at the initial visit including issues of delivery mode, breastfeeding (not recommended for infants born to women living with HIV), contraception, and infant antiretroviral treatment. Although these issues do not need to be fully resolved at the initial visit, early introduction allows time for discussion and planning.

A comprehensive review of the medical history is routine for all women. For women living with HIV, this history should include an expanded history related to HIV and its management. This includes viral load, CD4, HIV-associated opportunistic infections, need for prophylaxis for opportunistic infection, routine infectious/STI screening augmented with hepatitis A and tuberculosis, and assessment of need for vaccination for hepatitis A, hepatitis B, influenza, pneumococcus, and Tdap. Additional laboratory testing may include liver and renal function testing, HLA-B*5701 testing, and, as noted, antiretroviral drug resistance genotype testing if not already done.

Antiretroviral Use in Pregnancy

As a general statement, antiretroviral treatment in pregnancy follows the same guidelines as for nonpregnant patients. Beginning with a discussion of the risks and benefits of therapy, women living with HIV should be informed of the risk of disease progression, the risk of transmission to partners and the infant, the impact of therapy on transmission risk, the importance of adherence throughout all phases of the pregnancy (and lifelong), the known risks associated with proposed antiretroviral medications, and the limited data available regarding infant outcomes related to antiretroviral medications.

Specific medication selection is best done with the input of an expert in HIV management as recommendations may change with the introduction of new medication options. However, a few general principles apply to the selection of an appropriate antiretroviral regimen:

- As is true for the selection of all medications, side effects, cost, convenience, interaction with other medications and prior experience with the proposed medication impact selection.
- Regimens recommended for nonpregnant patients should be used for pregnant patients unless known risk outweighs benefit. The corollary to this is that women on fully suppressive therapy at the time of presentation should, generally, continue that regimen.

- Pregnancy-related physiologic changes may alter the pharmacokinetics of anti-retroviral therapy requiring close monitoring of viral load and possible adjust-ment of dose.
- One current antiretroviral medication, dolutegravir, has specific pregnancy-related recommendations. It is not recommended for use in the first trimester as it is associated with an increased risk for neural tube defects. It may be used after the first trimester. Patients taking dolutegravir and presenting for care should receive counseling regarding known and possible risks of each option including continuation of therapy, discontinuation of therapy, and changing therapy.

Intrapartum Management

As is true in preconception and prenatal period, management of HIV in the intrapar-tum period should largely consist of the established antiretroviral regimen. Conversely, in the presence of adequate antiretroviral therapy, intrapartum manage-ment of patients living with HIV is similar in most ways to the management of other laboring patients. In addition to continuing the antepartum antiretroviral regimen, there may be a role for the addition of zidovudine during labor or cesarean section. The decision to add zidovudine is based on the viral load at the time of delivery. For patients with a viral load that is undetectable and for whom adherence with antiret-roviral therapy has been good, no zidovudine is necessary. Zidovudine may be used for patients with a detectable viral load less than 1000 or when adherence to antiret-roviral therapy is unknown or incomplete. For those patients with a viral load above 1000, zidovudine is recommended.

For patients with a viral load at or above 1000, a scheduled cesarean section at 38 weeks is recommended to reduce the risk of perinatal transmission. This is in addition to the use of IV zidovudine in this setting. It should be noted that the rec-ommendation for cesarean delivery assumes a scheduled c-section in a non-laboring patient with intact membranes. There is insufficient evidence to determine the ben-efit of cesarean delivery either for patients who present in active labor or for patients who present with rupture of membranes.

For women with viral loads <1000, routine decisions regarding cesarean section should be based on factors other than perinatal transmission. The rate of transmis-sion is low for all patients in this group and is not improved with the routine use of cesarean delivery.

In the absence of antiretroviral therapy, every effort should be made to reduce intrapartum procedures. In patients who are adequately treated with antiretroviral therapy and without evidence of viremia, artificial rupture of membranes may be performed if indicated. Fetal scalp electrodes and assisted delivery (forceps or vacuum-assisted device) should be avoided unless clearly indicated. Data regarding transmission associated with episiotomy is limited.

Antiretroviral therapy can impact pharmacologic intervention in postpartum hemorrhage management. Antiretroviral therapy that inhibits cytochrome P450 3A4 is a relative contraindication to the use of Methergine unless no alternative exists. Antiretroviral therapy that induces cytochrome P450 3A4 may decrease the efficacy of uterotonic agents (due to decreased Methergine availability).

Postpartum Management

Postpartum management of patients living with HIV is similar in most ways to the management of all postpartum patients with a few notable exceptions. Breastfeeding is not recommended in the United States for patients with known HIV infection. This recommendation is not impacted by viral load or the use of antiretroviral therapy.

Maternal antiretroviral therapy should be continued uninterrupted. As the postpartum period offers many barriers to adherence, these should be proactively addressed with the mother and her support system. As noted above, the management of HIV in pregnancy is more ideal when the pregnancy is planned. For this reason postpartum care should include discussion of a contraceptive plan prior to discharge from the hospital and reviewed at subsequent postpartum office visits.

In general, antiretroviral therapy regimens will not have been changed to accommodate pregnancy. If they have been changed, plans regarding any post-pregnancy therapy changes should be coordinated to ensure continuity and should reflect best practice for nonpregnant adults.

All newborns of women living with HIV should receive antiretroviral therapy following delivery. The regimen, duration, and follow-up should be directed by providers familiar with the management of HIV in infants.

Chapter 18
Multigestational Pregnancy

Contents

Background.. 149
Diagnosis... 151
  History... 152
  Physical Examination.. 152
  Laboratory and Diagnostic Studies.. 152
Management... 152
  Prenatal Care.. 152
  Labor and Delivery... 153

> **Key Points**
> 1. Multigestational pregnancy presents unique management challenges beyond those encountered in singleton pregnancies.
> 2. Multigestational pregnancy may result from either a single or multiple fertilized ovum (ova).
> 3. Complications associated with multigestational pregnancies include spontaneous abortion, preterm delivery, pre-eclampsia, postpartum hemorrhage, and increased perinatal mortality.

Background

Most pregnancies are the product of a single fertilized ovum and result in a single fetus. One to two percent of pregnancies, however, result in multiple fetuses, multigestational pregnancy. Such pregnancies present unique challenges for both prenatal management and delivery. Although uncommon, multigestational pregnancy occurs with sufficient frequency that primary care providers should be familiar with basic management considerations.

© Springer Nature Switzerland AG 2020

P. Lyons, N. McLaughlin, *Obstetrics in Family Medicine*, Current Clinical Practice,
https://doi.org/10.1007/978-3-030-39888-0_18

   Multiple gestations may be the result of either a single fertilized ovum that divides early in development or multiple fertilized ova from the same cycle. Monozygotic (MZ) twins are genetically identical fetuses produced from a single fertilized ovum. MZ twins make up about 30% of all twin pregnancies. Dizygotic (DZ) twins are the product of two separate fertilized ova. Although they are genetically similar, they are not genetically identical. DZ twins make up 70% of all twin pregnancies with a frequency of approximately 1 out of 80 pregnancies. Although significantly less common, multigestational pregnancy may result in more than two developing fetuses. The expected natural frequency of multigestational pregnancy is approximately 1 in 80 twins, 1 in 6400 triplets, and 1 in 512,000 quadruplets. The increase in assisted fertility has significantly altered the frequency of multigestational pregnancies, however, and such figures may no longer be entirely applicable.

   In addition to multiple fetuses, multigestational pregnancies may have several variations of multiple chorions and placentae. MZ twins may have a single placenta and a single chorion (~60%) or may have two chorions with either a fused placenta or two separate placentae (~20% each). DZ twins have two chorions and two placentae, which may be fused or separate (~50% each).

   Multigestational pregnancies are associated with increased risk for a variety of prenatal and delivery-related complications (*see* Table 18.1). Maternal risks associated with multigestational pregnancy include spontaneous abortion, stillbirth, preterm labor, preterm delivery, placental previa, anemia, urinary tract infection (UTI), pre-eclampsia, and postpartum hemorrhage. Up to two-thirds of twin pregnancies will result in loss of one twin in the first trimester. The rate of fetal demise is twice

Table 18.1 Complications of multigestational pregnancy

Maternal complications
Spontaneous abortion
Stillbirth
Preterm labor
Preterm delivery
Placenta previa
Gestational diabetes
Anemia
Urinary tract infection
Pregnancy-induced hypertension/pre-eclampsia
Postpartum hemorrhage
Fetal complications
Perinatal mortality
Developmental abnormalities
Growth abnormalities
Preterm delivery complications

as high as for single pregnancies. The risk of both anemia and UTI is 2–3 times normal. There is a threefold increased risk of pre-eclampsia and a fivefold increased risk of postpartum hemorrhage in multigestational pregnancy.

Fetal risks include developmental abnormalities, growth abnormalities, and preterm delivery complications, including a death rate that is three times the normal. Perinatal mortality is three times that of single pregnancy risk. The risk of both major and minor malformations is double that of single pregnancies. The average gestational age at delivery is 36 weeks for twins and 33 weeks for triplets, significantly increasing the likelihood of complications from prematurity.

Diagnosis

The diagnosis of multiple gestations is generally made via ultrasound (US) during the course of prenatal care. Careful prenatal care combined with the prevalence of obstetrical US has greatly diminished the number of unanticipated multigestational deliveries. Although the diagnosis is generally made ultrasonographically, the provider's index of suspicion may be heightened by historical or physical examination findings during the course of prenatal care. Key findings are summarized in Table 18.2.

Table 18.2 Findings associated with multigestation

History
Family history of multigestational pregnancy (including patients who are themselves twins)
Past history of multigestational pregnancy
Assisted reproduction
Maternal symptoms
Nausea
Vomiting
Headache
Shortness of breath
Abdominal distention
Constipation
Physical findings
Uterus size larger than dates
Excess maternal weight gain
Multiple palpable fetuses
Multiple audible fetal heart tones
Laboratory/diagnostic studies
Significantly decreased hemoglobin
Elevated maternal serum α-fetoprotein
Ultrasound documentation of multiple fetuses

History

Prior to conception or early in the prenatal course, a past history or family history of multigestational pregnancy should be explored. In addition, a history of assisted reproduction should be noted, when present. Patients with multigestational pregnancy may report an increase in pelvic pressure, nausea, vomiting, headache, shortness of breath, distention, and constipation. Although none of these symptoms is specific to multigestational pregnancy, the number of symptoms and/or the severity of the complaint may be increased in such pregnancies.

Physical Examination

Because the symptoms noted here are neither sensitive nor specific for multigestational pregnancy, suggestive physical findings may be important in identifying patients with multiple fetuses. Increased maternal weight gain is a nonspecific but suggestive finding. Uterine size greater than expected for gestational age may also be a critical finding. Two palpable fetuses or multiple fetal heart tones, although less common, should prompt immediate US evaluation.

Laboratory and Diagnostic Studies

As previously noted, obstetrical US is the definitive study. In skilled hands, US may demonstrate multiple gestations as early as 4 weeks' gestation. Other suggestive laboratory findings include decreased hemoglobin and elevated maternal serum α-fetoprotein (levels approximately 2–3 times higher than for singleton pregnancies even in the absence of fetal abnormalities).

Management

Prenatal Care

In general, the course of prenatal care is similar to that of singleton pregnancies with additional care directed toward specific increased risks associated with multigestational pregnancy. The diagnosis should be confirmed as early as possible. For patients at high risk (e.g., assisted reproduction), this may include US documentation as early as 4 weeks' gestation. Because of the increased potential for genetic abnormalities, providers may consider offering genetic diagnosis for patients over the age of 33. The frequency of prenatal visits may be increased to monitor for signs/symptoms of preterm contractions or preterm labor.

Patients should be counseled concerning the increased need for careful dietary intake. Folic acid supplementation should be started at the first prenatal visit, and iron supplementation may also be appropriate. Maternal weight gain should be closely monitored with a target weight gain of 35–45 lb over the course of pregnancy.

Fetal growth should be closely monitored starting early in the third trimester (or earlier if patient is determined to be at risk for abnormal fetal growth). US studies every 4 weeks will allow for documentation of adequate and symmetric fetal growth.

Labor and Delivery

Management of multigestational deliveries is associated with several significant challenges. Providers with limited experience or without access to necessary obstetrical and neonatal support should arrange for appropriate backup or transfer prior to the onset of labor. Patients with three or more fetuses are generally not candidates for vaginal delivery, and arrangements should be made early in the prenatal course for appropriate cesarean section.

Because the method of delivery may vary with the presentation of the infants at the time of labor, patients with twin pregnancies should be admitted at the first signs of labor, bleeding per vagina, or rupture of membranes. On admission, US should be performed to confirm the position and presentation of each infant. All twin deliveries should be attended by one pediatric team (with all necessary neonatal resuscitation equipment) for each infant.

By convention, the first twin is designated twin A and the second, twin B. Possible variations of presentation include (a) twin A vertex, twin B vertex (~40%), (b) twin A vertex, twin B breech (~40%), or (c) twin A breech, twin B any presentation (~20%). Vaginal delivery can only be attempted if twin A is in a vertex presentation; therefore, pregnancies with twin A in a breech position at the time of labor will require cesarean section delivery. If twin A is in a vertex presentation at the time of labor and there are no other contraindications, vaginal delivery may be attempted. In addition to the usual indications for cesarean section associated with any pregnancy (*see* Chap. 22), cesarean section is indicated in twin deliveries that demonstrate twin–twin transfusion.

Because the position of twin B cannot be absolutely known prior to delivery of twin A, all attempted vaginal deliveries should be performed in a setting equipped for a cesarean section if necessary. All patients should have intravenous access, available typed and crossmatched blood, and a complete blood count prior to delivery.

Vaginal delivery of the first twin is managed in a similar manner to singleton deliveries. Following the delivery of twin A, US should be performed to confirm the presentation of twin B. If twin B is in a vertex presentation, delivery is again managed in a manner similar to singleton pregnancies. If twin B is found to be in a breech position following delivery of twin A, external version may be attempted to position the infant in a vertex presentation. If twin B remains in a breech position, cesarean section should be performed.

Chapter 19
Postdates Pregnancy

Contents

Background.. 155
Diagnosis... 156
  History.. 156
  Physical Examination.. 157
  Diagnostic Studies.. 157
  Management.. 157
  Assessment of Fetal Well-Being.. 157
Fetal Kick Count... 158
Amniotic Fluid Volume.. 159
Ultrasound Estimate of Fetal Weight.. 159
Nonstress Test... 159
Contraction Stress Test.. 159
Biophysical Profile.. 160

Key Points
1. Term pregnancy is defined as 37–42 weeks' gestation.
2. Accurate pregnancy dating is critical to assessment and management of postdates pregnancy.
3. Timing of delivery should be prior to 42 weeks' gestation and earlier if antenatal testing is nonreassuring.

Background

When a firm estimated date of delivery (EDD) is established early in pregnancy, providers can anticipate that most pregnancies will result in spontaneous delivery at term. The incidence of delivery at or beyond 42 weeks is approximately 3:1000 pregnancies. Under some circumstances, however, pregnancy may continue beyond 42 weeks, requiring assessment and management as a postdates pregnancy. The

© Springer Nature Switzerland AG 2020
P. Lyons, N. McLaughlin, *Obstetrics in Family Medicine*, Current Clinical Practice,
https://doi.org/10.1007/978-3-030-39888-0_19

cause of prolonged gestation is not well understood, but patients with one postterm delivery have a 50% likelihood of subsequent postterm delivery.

A significant first step in identifying postdates pregnancies is confirmation of gestational dating. As noted in Chap. 3, a variety of measurements may be used to establish the EDD, including the last menstrual period (LMP) and obstetrical ultrasound (US). Confirmation of the EDD is critical to appropriate management of postdates pregnancy. For this reason, all such data should be reviewed carefully and confirmed.

Although pregnancy is not considered postdates until 42 weeks of gestation, planning for management should begin at or near the EDD. Careful fetal monitoring and management for delivery is critical as postdates pregnancy is associated with an increased risk for operative delivery, macrosomia, shoulder dystocia, meconium aspiration, and fetal mortality (twice baseline at 42 weeks, six times baseline by 44 weeks).

Diagnosis

Studies suggest that accurate dating may reduce prevalence of postdates pregnancy by almost half. That would make inaccurate dating the most common "cause" of postdates pregnancy. For this reason, confirmation of the appropriate gestational age is critical. In general, dating is based on the patient's report of last menstrual period supported by ultrasound data.

History

The patient's menstrual history should be reviewed, including the timing and normality of the LMP. Under a variety of conditions, the episode of bleeding considered to be the LMP may be inaccurate. Oligomenorrhea, prior use of contraception such as oral contraception or medroxyprogesterone, and pregnancy-related first-trimester bleeding may all alter the accuracy of menstrual history. First-trimester bleeding per vagina is very common, and such bleeding may be interpreted as menstrual bleeding when, in fact, it was not. Early pregnancy bleeding is reviewed in Chap. 9.

The date of the first positive pregnancy test may be helpful in narrowing the possible dates of pregnancy. A review of the prenatal record should include obstetrical US results, if available, fundal height measurements, fetal quickening, and first noted fetal heart tones by US (4–6 weeks), handheld Doppler (10–12 weeks), or fetoscope (18–20 weeks). A pelvic examination with bimanual assessment of uterine size early in pregnancy may also provide confirmatory support for EDD.

Prior obstetrical history should be reviewed as a past history of postdates delivery is associated with an increased risk of subsequent postdates delivery.

Physical Examination

Primary confirmation of postdates pregnancy is generally provided by a careful history. Physical examination is generally supplementary at term and should not alter an otherwise well-established EDD.

Diagnostic Studies

In the absence of adequate prenatal data to establish EDD, late-pregnancy US may provide a broad estimate of gestational age. US accuracy diminishes with increasing gestational age, however, and late-pregnancy results should be interpreted with caution. Although the exact accuracy of dating by US cannot be established, the "1 week per trimester" rule of thumb is a reasonable estimate of accuracy. US studies performed in the first trimester are accurate to within 1 week; those performed in the second are accurate to within 2 weeks; those performed in the third trimester are accurate to within 3 weeks. If the dating by ultrasound varies by more than this limit, ultrasound data should be used to establish the EDD. If dating by ultrasound varies by less than this limit, EDD should be based on LMP.

Management

Postdates pregnancy presents two related challenges to providers: (a) assessment of continued fetal well-being and (b) assessment of need for induction.

Induction of labor is discussed in Chap. 20. As a general rule, the risk associated with postdates pregnancy after 42 weeks' gestation provides support for a policy of induction at or before that time. An overview of management is provided in Fig. 19.1.

Assessment of Fetal Well-Being

A variety of tests to assess fetal well-being are available. These tests range from patient-performed outpatient monitoring to formal monitoring with US examination. Prenatal care providers should be familiar with each of these options, their role in the management of postdates pregnancy, and the strengths and limitations of each study. Assessment of fetal well-being should begin between 40 and 41 weeks of gestation and should continue until delivery.

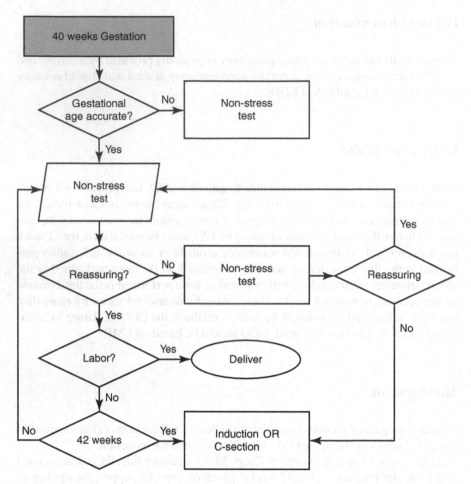

Fig. 19.1 Management of postdates pregnancy

Fetal Kick Count

Thirty to 60 minutes postprandial, lying on her left side, the patient monitors and counts fetal movements ("kicks"). Normal frequency is approximately five kicks per hour. Fewer than ten kicks in 2 h is considered abnormal. Although a reasonable adjunct to other methods of monitoring, fetal kick counts alone are probably insufficient to ensure fetal well-being. All reports of decreased fetal movement should be followed up by a nonstress test (NST) or a biophysical profile.

Amniotic Fluid Volume

Amniotic fluid volume can be calculated weekly. Although not a direct measure of fetal well-being, oligohydramnios (low fluid volume) is an indication for delivery. Because the result of this test may alter clinical management, amniotic fluid volume has become standard practice.

Ultrasound Estimate of Fetal Weight

Like the amniotic fluid volume, assessment of fetal weight is not a direct measure of fetal well-being. However, just as with amniotic fluid volume, the outcome of the study may impact management and is therefore commonly included in the assessment of postdates pregnancies. Although ultrasound estimates of fetal weight are subject to an error of up to 500 g, estimated fetal weight may alter delivery planning. Macrosomia is an indication for possible elective caesarian section (5000 g in nondiabetic patients; 4500 g in patients with diabetes).

Nonstress Test

During the NST, patients are monitored with external to codynamometer and a Doppler fetal heart rate monitor. A reassuring NST consists of at least two accelerations in fetal heart rate in 15–20 min. Each acceleration should last at least 15 s and increase at least 15 beats per minute from baseline. (Fetal heart rate monitoring is reviewed in Chap. 26.) Nonstress testing should be repeated twice weekly beginning at 40–41 weeks' gestation.

Nonreassuring NSTs may be associated with threats to fetal well-being, may represent a period of fetal sleep, or may be related to external factors such as medication. Nonreassuring NSTs should prompt additional follow-up.

Contraction Stress Test

Fetal stimulation associated with uterine contraction has been observed to induce decelerations of fetal heart rate in circumstances where fetal well-being is threatened. This observation led to the development of the contraction stress test. Oxytocin is used to induce uterine contractions. The fetal heart rate is monitored, in turn, for decelerations indicative of fetal stress. Contraindications to contraction stress test include preterm labor risk, classical cesarean section scar, and placenta previa.

Oxytocin is started at 0.5–1.0 mU per minute and increased every 15 min until a pattern of three contractions every 10 min is established. Late decelerations with 50% or more of contractions are considered a positive test and require further evaluation. Infrequent late decelerations should prompt close monitoring and possible further evaluation. Variable decelerations should be followed by US evaluation to assess amniotic fluid status. A normal or negative test (no late or variable decelerations) is reassuring and should prompt routine fetal monitoring.

Biophysical Profile

A biophysical profile is a multicomponent assessment of fetal well-being. Each of the five components is given a score of 0–2 with a maximum possible score of 10. A score of 8 is reassuring; 6 is suspicious; 4 indicates a need for acute intervention.

The scoring matrix is summarized in Table 19.1. Components of the biophysical profile include the following:

1. An NST is performed. A reassuring NST is scored 2. A nonreassuring NST is scored 0.
2. Amniotic fluid index (AFI) score is obtained. An AFI score of 5 or higher with at least one 2 cm × 2 cm pocket of amniotic fluid present is scored 2 points. AFI less than 5 or no pocket of fluid is scored 0.
3. Sustained fetal breathing is monitored. Sustained fetal breathing of at least 30 s is scored 2. Absence of fetal breathing activity or duration less than 30 s is scored 0.
4. Fetal movement is monitored. At least three limb or trunk movements are scored 2. Less than three movements is scored 0.
5. Fetal tone is measured. Fetus flexion at rest with at least one movement of extension followed by return to flexion is scored 2. Extension at rest or lack of at least one extension/flexion movement is scored 0.

Table 19.1 Biophysical profile scoring

Measure	Normal (2 points)	Abnormal (0 points)
Amniotic fluid	At least one pocket ≥2 cm	No pocket ≥2 cm
Fetal heart rate	Reactive two or more episodes; acceleration (≥15 beats per minute over baseline) lasting at least 15 s within 20 min	Nonreactive
Fetal tone	Active limb extension and flexion	Slow extension, no return to flexion, no movement or partially open fetal hand
Gross movement	At least two separate limb or body movements within 30 min	Fewer than two separate limb or body movements within 30 min
Breathing movements	At least one episode lasting >20 s within 30 min	No episode of sufficient duration within 30 min

Part III
Labor and Delivery

Chapter 20
Normal Labor

Contents

Background.. 163
Prelabor... 164
Labor.. 164
Assessment.. 165
   History.. 165
   Physical Examination... 165
Dilation... 166
Effacement.. 166
Station.. 166
Presentation... 166
Laboratory Studies.. 167
Management.. 167

Key Points
1. Labor is defined as uterine contractions resulting in progressive cervical change.
2. Assessment of labor begins with confirmation of gestational age.

Background

The experience of labor and delivery is the culmination of the prenatal period. It is the period with the most potential for both the most joy and the most anxiety.

© Springer Nature Switzerland AG 2020
P. Lyons, N. McLaughlin, *Obstetrics in Family Medicine*, Current Clinical Practice,
https://doi.org/10.1007/978-3-030-39888-0_20

Prelabor

Prior to labor there is generally a sequence of predictable events that mark the physiological preparation for delivery of the infant. Beginning 4–8 weeks prior to delivery, the patient may begin to experience slight, irregular, and non-sustained contractions. These contractions, referred to as Braxton Hicks, are marked by only mild discomfort in most circumstances and do not lead to cervical change.

Approximately 2 weeks prior to delivery, the fetal head will often settle into the pelvic brim. This settling is referred to as lightening, and the patient may report that the baby has "dropped." There is potentially a measurable decrease in fundal height, and the patient may report a decrease in pregnancy symptoms related to intra-abdominal pressure. The woman may also, however, report an increase in symptoms related to fetal pressure within the pelvis.

Beginning several days to several weeks prior to delivery, the cervix will begin to undergo preparatory changes that will include softening and may also include some degree of effacement and dilation. Dilation up to 3 cm may occur during this phase and is generally more pronounced in multiparous patients. A standardized measure of cervical condition exists and is often used in the evaluation of patients for possible induction of labor, when necessary. The Bishop scale is summarized in Table 20.1.

As the cervix begins to dilate and efface, the cervical mucus plug that has occupied the os during the course of pregnancy comes out. This is occasionally associated with a small amount of blood referred to as "bloody show." The loss of the mucus plug and bloody show are generally signs that the onset of labor is imminent.

Labor

Labor is divided into three separate stages, which are summarized in Table 20.2. The first stage of labor is from the onset of contractions through full cervical dilation and effacement. Because the early cervical changes may be protracted and

Table 20.1 Bishop scale cervical scoring

	Score			
Indicator	0	1	2	3
Dilation (cm)	0	1–2	3–4	5–6
Effacement (%)	0–30	40–50	60–80	80–100
Fetal station	−3	−2	−1/0	≥ + 1
Consistency	Firm	Medium	Soft	
Cervical position	Posterior	Mid	Anterior	

Table 20.2 Stages of labor

First stage	Onset to full dilation	Primigravid, 6–18 h (mean, 12)	1.2 cm/h	Effacement, dilation, station
		Multiparous, 2–10 h (mean, 6.5)	1.5 cm/h	
Second stage	Full dilation to delivery of infant	Primigravid, 1–3 h		Descent, rotation
		Multiparous, 5–30 min		
Third stage	Delivery of infant to delivery of placenta	Up to 30 min		Delivery of placenta

unpredictable in their course, the first stage of labor is divided into early- or latent-phase labor and active-phase labor. Although no absolute distinction can be made between these two phases of the first stage of labor, patients are generally considered in latent-phase labor until cervical dilation reaches approximately 6 cm. The second stage of labor begins with full cervical dilation and continues until delivery of the infant. The third stage of labor begins with the delivery of the infant and is complete with the delivery of the placenta. Although the duration of each stage is highly variable, the duration tends to shorten with each subsequent pregnancy.

Assessment

History

Assessment of possible labor begins with an abbreviated history. Accurate pregnancy dating is critical to the appropriate management of labor. If uncertain dating makes preterm labor a possibility, the patient must be managed as if preterm. A complete discussion of the management can be found in Chap. 7. In addition to gestational dating, the history should include a review of the prenatal course and any complications that arose during pregnancy. Pre-existing medical conditions, including any allergies, should be reviewed. A history of the contractions should include onset, frequency, duration, and intensity. Patients should be asked about bleeding or rupture of membranes. Fetal movement should be confirmed.

Physical Examination

Physical examination should include vital signs, abdominal examination of the abdomen including Leopold's maneuvers, and a clinical estimate of fetal size. A manual examination of the cervix should be performed to determine dilation, effacement, station, and presentation.

Dilation

Cervical dilation is measured in centimeters and ranges from 0 (closed) to 10 (complete). Standardized instruments exist that allow providers to "feel" various degrees of dilation, and providers should occasionally test their own assessment against these instruments. Hand size varies significantly, but 1 cm dilation is approximately equivalent to a fingertip. A measurement of 3 cm is approximately equivalent to two fingers side by side. A 5 cm dilation is approximately equivalent to spreading index and middle fingers in a "victory" sign, and 10 cm is roughly equivalent to fully spread index and middle fingers. Complete dilation to 10 cm might alternatively be thought of as the absence of appreciable cervical tissue on exam.

Effacement

Effacement represents thinning of the cervix over the fetal head (or presenting body part in non-vertex presentations). This can be visualized as equivalent to pulling a tight turtleneck sweater over one's head. Effacement is described in percentages, with 0% effacement marking no change and 100% effacement representing no appreciable thickness to the cervix. Although dilation and effacement often occur in tandem, either may occur without evidence of the other.

Station

Station refers to the position of the fetal head in the birth canal. Zero station is defined as the level of the ischial spines. Positions above the ischial spines are measured as negative values, whereas positions below the ischial spines are measured as positive values. Traditionally, the distances were divided in thirds. A fetal head is one-third of the distance between the ischial spines, and the outlet is +1, two-thirds +2, and at the outlet +3. The same applies in reverse for negative station measures. Some authorities now recommend measuring in centimeters from the spines, which translates to a −6 to +6 scale. Considerable head molding may occur during descent, and providers should be careful to measure distance to the fetal head and not to the fetal caput.

Presentation

During the examination, the presenting body part should be examined and confirmed. If a cephalic (head-first) presentation cannot be confirmed on manual examination, an ultrasound should be performed.

Laboratory Studies

Prenatal labs should be reviewed, and any missing laboratory values should be ordered. In particular, hemoglobin, platelets, and evidence of infection (including group B strep) should be noted. Additional labs may be required if the patient is presenting with a complication of pregnancy or labor.

Management

In the first stage of labor, management is generally expectant. Patients should be admitted (preferably as late in the first stage as possible under most circumstances). Blood pressure should be checked every 2–4 h, and fetal heart rate should be monitored every 30 min, unless abnormalities arise. Patients may be allowed to ambulate, but intake by mouth should be limited. Adequate anesthesia should be provided at the request of the patient. Recent studies support the use of early anesthesia if requested by the patient.

The second stage of labor is marked by descent of the fetal head through the birth canal. The usual sequence of head movements is engagement, flexion, descent, internal rotation, extension, external rotation, and expulsion.

Delivery will usually occur without any necessary assistance on the part of the provider. At the time of delivery of the head, gentle counterpressure may be applied to control delivery and minimize perineal trauma. Delivery of the anterior shoulder is effected with gentle downward traction followed by delivery of the posterior shoulder in an upward motion.

With delivery of the head, a quick check is made to ensure that no nuchal cord is present, and bulb suction of the infant's nose and mouth should be performed. The mother should breathe rather than push during this activity. With delivery of the body, the infant should be placed on the maternal abdomen, dried, and stimulated; cord clamping should be delayed 30–60 s, unless medical attention is needed for the newborn or the mother.

Delivery of the placenta also requires little assistance from the provider under normal circumstances. Gentle traction on the umbilical cord may assist with release, but excess traction may lead to uterine inversion, or cord rupture, and excess postpartum hemorrhage. The delivering provider should observe for the signs of placental separation; fundal elevation, cord prolongation, and a gush of blood.

Chapter 21
Induction and Augmentation

Contents

Background... 169
Preparation.. 169
   Pharmacological Options.. 170
   Mechanical Options.. 171
Induction.. 171

> **Key Points**
> 1. Induction is defined as artificial initiation of labor.
> 2. Augmentation is defined as artificial stimulation of labor.
> 3. Induction should always be performed for a specific indication.

Background

Under most circumstances, the initiation of labor occurs without assistance at the appropriate time. Under some circumstances, however, induction of labor is indicated prior to the onset of labor via natural processes. Table 21.1 presents a list of indications for induction. Induction should always be performed for a specific indication and, when possible, under circumstances where cervical status is favorable for delivery.

Preparation

Prior to induction patients should be carefully assessed for contraindications to induction (*see* Table 21.2). In addition, cervical status should be assessed. A Bishop cervical score (*see* Chap. 18) of 8 predicts a success rate for induction approximately equivalent to spontaneous labor.

© Springer Nature Switzerland AG 2020
P. Lyons, N. McLaughlin, *Obstetrics in Family Medicine*, Current Clinical Practice,
https://doi.org/10.1007/978-3-030-39888-0_21

Table 21.1 Indications for induction

Preeclampsia
Chronic hypertension
Diabetes mellitus
Heart disease
Postdates
Rh incompatibility
Fetal abnormalities or demise
Chorioamnionitis
Premature rupture of membranes
Intrauterine growth restriction

Table 21.2 Contraindications to induction of labor

Pelvic abnormalities incompatible with vaginal delivery
Placenta previa
Classical cesarean section scar
Full-thickness myomectomy
Hysterotomy
Breech presentation not compatible with vaginal delivery

If the cervical status is not favorable for induction and the need for delivery is not immediate, cervical preparation may be a helpful adjunct in preparing for delivery. Several modalities are available to enhance favorable cervical status, including mechanical and pharmacological options.

Pharmacological Options

Prostaglandin formulations are available including PGE1 (misoprostol) and PGE2 (dinoprostone). Both mimic the prostaglandin activity physiologically present with the onset of spontaneous labor. Misoprostol is available as a pill that can be placed intravaginally or orally (buccally) (25 µg every 3–6 h). Dinoprostone is available in a gel formulation (0.5 mg/2.5 mg gel). A single dose is placed intracervically and can be repeated in 6–12 h. Contraindications to prostaglandin use include unexplained bleeding per vagina, rupture of membranes, and prior cesarean section. In addition to those general contraindications, dinoprostone should be used with caution in patients with a history of asthma and is contraindicated in patients with glaucoma or a history of myocardial infarction. Side effects include fetal stress and decelerations, hypertonicity, nausea, vomiting, and fever.

Mechanical Options

Two mechanical options are also available for cervical ripening. These are placement of a Foley bulb and hygroscopic dilators (laminaria). A Foley catheter with a 25–50 cc balloon may be inserted above the internal os, inflated, and withdrawn to the internal os. Within 12 h, the cervix can be expected to dilate 2–3 cm. This dilation will be apparent clinically when the Foley bulb falls out of the cervix. The laminaria is placed in the cervix, and as the fluid is absorbed, the laminaria swells to three to four times its original size within 6–12 h.

Preparation for induction should also include preparation for failure of induction and therefore should only be performed in a setting where access to operative delivery is available.

Induction

Induction is generally performed with oxytocin. Specific protocols vary between institutions, and providers should be aware of the specific protocol at their own institution. One potential regimen is 10 units of oxytocin in 1 L of fluid. The oxytocin is attached to an infusion pump and is slowly titrated up until adequate contractions are achieved or contraindications to continue induction develop. Complications include hyperstimulation with possible tetanic contractions, abruptio placentae, uterine rupture, precipitous delivery, cord prolapse, and fetal stress. Because of the potential serious nature of these side effects, patients must have vital signs monitored regularly and must have both fetal heart rate and tocodynamometer monitoring during the course of induction. Details of fetal heart rate monitoring are reviewed in Chap. 28.

Chapter 22
Pain Management in Labor

Contents

Background.. 173
Nonpharmacological Management... 174
Pharmacological Management.. 174
   Narcotic Analgesia.. 174
   Local Anesthesia... 175
   Epidural–Spinal Anesthesia.. 175

> **Key Points**
> 1. Pain in labor is a multifaceted experience with physiological, psychological, and social components.
> 2. Pain management in labor requires a multifaceted approach, including pharmacological and nonpharmacological options.
> 3. Appropriate pain management will greatly enhance the experience of labor.

Background

Virtually all labor is accompanied by pain. Uterine contractions, cervical dilation, fetal descent, and perineal stretching (and, when it occurs, laceration) are all associated with pain. Although pain accompanies all labor, the patient's perception of and response to pain is highly variable. Providers must be aware of all factors that contribute to the patient's pain and adequately address each of these factors in order to achieve appropriate pain control.

Although the patient's perception of pain depends on a variety of factors, the physiological basis of pain is reasonably well described. In the first stage of labor, most pain is secondary to uterine contractions, intermittent ischemia, and cervical dilation. The primary neurological innervation associated with these components is

P. Lyons, N. McLaughlin, *Obstetrics in Family Medicine*, Current Clinical Practice,
https://doi.org/10.1007/978-3-030-39888-0_22

located at the level of T10–L1. In the second stage of labor, vaginal and perineal distentions are the primary source of pain. Innervation is at the level of S2–S4, the pudendal nerve.

Options for pain management include pharmacological and nonpharmacological modalities with which providers should be familiar. Among the nonpharmacological options are hydrotherapy, hypnotherapy, positioning, and support. Pharmacological options include epidural–spinal anesthesia, narcotic pain management, and local anesthesia.

Nonpharmacological Management

Ideally, nonpharmacological modalities are a part of the management of all labor. Such management begins in the prenatal period with appropriate education concerning the process of labor and delivery and a discussion of reasonable expectations concerning pain in labor. In addition, patients will often benefit from a prenatal course in one of the many nonpharmacological approaches to pain management.

Although the specifics of each approach vary somewhat, several key principles are shared among all approaches. These principles include relaxation, suggestion, concentration, and preparation. With appropriate preparation and intrapartum support, the efficacy of nonpharmacological approaches is quite high, approaching 80% in some populations.

Patients should be educated concerning the duration of each stage of labor, the expected events of each stage, and the active role that laboring mothers have in contributing to the success of each stage. Patients should receive education concerning preadmission management of pain, appropriate timing of presentation to the labor and delivery suite, and warning symptoms that require prompt assessment.

At the time of labor, patients are counseled to anticipate contractions, to focus on each contraction in turn, to develop a point of focus for each contraction, and to use relaxation techniques including visualization and breathing techniques. As with all skills, practice is an important component of the success of this technique, and introduction should begin early in the course of pregnancy to allow for adequate preparation.

Pharmacological Management

Narcotic Analgesia

Narcotic analgesics are nonspecific agents for pain management and can be successfully utilized for pain management in labor. Narcotics, in general, cross the placenta and will affect the fetus as well as the mother. Fetal side effects may include sedation and respiratory depression. Narcotic analgesia should be used with caution late in the course of the first stage of labor to minimize these side effects in the newborn. All delivery suites should have ready access to naloxone for use in infants with evidence of narcotic-related side effects at the time of delivery.

A variety of analgesic options are available for use in labor, and the specific agents used will vary from one institution to another. Providers should be familiar with the commonly employed agents at their institution. Among the acceptable agents commonly used in labor are nalbuphine 10–20 mg, typically given intravenously or intramuscularly, and butorphanol 1–2 mg IV/IM. Other newer opiates, including fentanyl, can be considered for their rapid onset and shorter duration of action.

Local Anesthesia

A variety of local anesthetic options are available and may be utilized during the course of labor. Local anesthesia is also often used postpartum prior to repair of lacerations or episiotomies. Commonly used options include tetracaine, lidocaine, and bupivacaine.

Epidural–Spinal Anesthesia

The most commonly employed pharmacological pain management modality in the United States is epidural or combined epidural–spinal anesthesia. Approximately 60% of all laboring patients receive such anesthesia. Epidural anesthesia provides improved pain control compared to systemic opiate pain medication. Epidural anesthesia involves introduction of pharmacological agents directly into the lumbar epidural space via a specialized needle and catheter system. Combination of epidural–spinal anesthesia involves epidural anesthesia along with the use of medication delivered to the subarachnoid space usually as a single dose. This bolus allows for relatively rapid effect. The addition of an epidural catheter allows for continued pain management over the course of labor, which as previously noted may be protracted. A significant benefit of the combined approach is the ability of the patient to ambulate for a longer time period than with epidural anesthesia alone.

Epidural anesthesia is delivered via catheter placed at the L3–L4 epidural space. The appropriate landmarks are identified, and a long epidural needle is introduced to the epidural space. A hollow needle is introduced first, followed by placement of the epidural catheter through the needle. The needle is then withdrawn and the catheter remains in place. Medication can be delivered continuously and/or as individual boluses through the catheter. Medication often includes a combination of analgesic and anesthetic agents.

Combination therapy involves introduction of the epidural needle followed by placement of a spinal needle into the subarachnoid space. A bolus of medication is delivered to the subarachnoid space. The spinal needle is withdrawn, the epidural catheter is placed, the epidural needle is withdrawn, and epidural anesthesia may follow as needed via the epidural catheter.

Patients should be closely monitored for changes in blood pressure, as hypotension is the most common complication of regional analgesia, and all patients should be on fetal heart rate monitors and tocodynamometers. Side effects associated with epidural anesthesia include maternal fever (which is probably not infectious in nature) and a 3% risk of placement in the subarachnoid space. Subarachnoid placement may be associated with postdural puncture headache. A growing body of high-quality evidence has demonstrated that early placement of epidural anesthesia does not appear to be related to delay in delivery or to an increased rate of cesarean section. Although local backache may be a transient side effect of epidural anesthesia, studies have shown no increase in long-term backache measured at 12 months' postpartum.

Part IV
Complications of Labor and Delivery

Chapter 23
Assisted Delivery

Contents

Background... 179
Forceps Delivery... 180
   Use of Forceps... 181
Vacuum-Assisted Delivery.. 181
Cesarean Section... 182

> ### Key Points
> 1. Assisted delivery is defined as any procedure undertaken to facilitate delivery of an infant.
> 2. Operative delivery methods include vacuum-assisted delivery, forceps delivery, and cesarean section.
> 3. Operative delivery should be undertaken for specific indications, and those indications should be specifically noted in labor record.

Background

Although most deliveries will result in spontaneous vaginal delivery, under some circumstances, additional assistance is required to deliver the infant. Assisted delivery is defined as any procedure undertaken to facilitate the delivery of the infant. These procedures may include vacuum-assisted delivery, use of forceps, and cesarean delivery. Indications for assisted delivery include prolonged second stage of labor (with adequate contractile force and documented insufficient progress), maternal factors that limit or preclude pushing or vaginal delivery (e.g., active genital herpes infection or vasa previa), fetal factors, or maternal medical problems indicating the need for urgent delivery. When present, these factors should be noted in the medical record and referenced in documentation of decision-making regarding assisted delivery.

© Springer Nature Switzerland AG 2020   179
P. Lyons, N. McLaughlin, *Obstetrics in Family Medicine*, Current Clinical Practice,
https://doi.org/10.1007/978-3-030-39888-0_23

Although each method has a role and each can be an important part of delivery management, each is different in success rate and complications. Specific comparison of forceps delivery with vacuum assist demonstrated a higher success rate with forceps but also a higher rate of high-grade (third and fourth degree) lacerations. Each method is associated with an injury pattern that reflects where and how the device is applied. Vacuum-assisted delivery may result in trauma in the area of the vacuum device—cephalohematoma, scalp injury, and retinal hemorrhage. The use of forceps is associated with a higher rate of facial injuries to the newborn.

There is no difference in the overall neonatal outcomes with no difference in Apgar scores, intubation, severe morbidity, or death. Likewise the rate of shoulder dystocia is the same with both methods.

Forceps Delivery

The use of forceps has become increasingly less common in obstetrics and is now relatively uncommon. The use of forceps, however, remains a critical skill in modern obstetrics, and a familiarity with the indications and general use of forceps is important for all providers of obstetrical care. The use of forceps should always be preceded by an assessment of the risks and benefits measured against the possibility of a cesarean section. Because of the skill and experience required to effectively utilize forceps and the potential complications associated with inappropriate use, forceps delivery should only be attempted for specific indications, when superior alternatives are not available or have been attempted, and by a provider with experience in both the identified indication and the appropriate use of forceps.

A variety of forceps models exist, and providers should be familiar with the available types and the indications for their use. In general, all forceps consist of two pieces with curved blades and locking handles. The curve of the blades is designed to accommodate the fetal head and the maternal pelvis. The blades are not interchangeable and must be positioned correctly to assist with the two principle activities of traction and fetal rotation.

Complications associated with the use of forceps include extension of the episiotomy, laceration, uterine or bladder rupture, transient facial paralysis, and intracranial damage.

The use of forceps is classified in part on the position of the infant in the birth canal. Historically, forceps have been used with fetuses in a variety of positions and in varying degrees of descent in the birth canal. Modern use of forceps is primarily limited to two areas, outlet forceps use and low forceps use.

Outlet forceps is defined as the use of forceps for an infant that is crowning with the skull at the pelvic floor. In addition, the position of the infant head must be identified with the sagittal suture in the anterior–posterior, right–left occiput anterior, or right–left occiput posterior positions. The use of outlet forceps should be limited to no more than 45° of fetal rotation.

Low forceps is defined as the use of forceps for an infant whose skull has reached at least +2 stations but that is not yet at the pelvic floor. Because low forceps use is, by definition, associated with less advanced infant progression through the birth canal, delivery may be associated with either less than or more than 45° of rotation.

Indications for forceps delivery include failure to progress with a prolonged second stage of labor, maternal cardiac or pulmonary disease, or nonreassuring fetal heart tracings. As previously noted, however, each of these indications should be considered in relation to the possibility of cesarean section as an alternative to forceps use.

Use of Forceps

Prior to the use of forceps, providers must first assess the adequacy of labor, maternal pelvic adequacy, and fetal position and station and must identify the specific indication for forceps use. There must be adequate uterine contractions and no evidence of cephalopelvic disproportion, and the fetal head must be at or below +2 stations with an appropriate presentation.

The steps involved in the use of forceps to effect forceps delivery are as follows:

1. Identify specific indication.
2. Rule out contraindications to forceps delivery, including assessment of maternal pelvic adequacy (ischial spine prominence, sacral contour, and suprapubic arch size).
3. Assess risks and benefits of cesarean section as an alternative.
4. Determine fetal head presentation.
5. Determine fetal head station.
6. Prepare for cesarean section in case of failed forceps delivery.
7. Place forceps appropriately.
8. Gentle traction and or rotation for delivery.

Vacuum-Assisted Delivery

The use of vacuum assist is similar to that of forceps. Providers should be aware that the use of vacuum assist rather than forceps does not alter the necessary steps prior to delivery. Although the mechanics of placement and delivery may appear to be less complex than for forceps delivery, vacuum-assisted delivery remains an operative delivery with associated risks and benefits and specific indications and contraindications.

A variety of vacuum-assisted devices exist, and providers should be familiar with the specific device utilized at their institution. In general, vacuum-assisted devices consist of a cup applied to the fetal head, a handle for providing traction, a mechanical or electric device for producing vacuum pressure, and a meter for measuring pressure.

Indications for vacuum-assisted delivery are similar to those for outlet forceps delivery. The nature of the vacuum-assisted device does not allow for fetal head rotation, and attempts to rotate the head may result in characteristic lacerations of the scalp. Contraindications to the use of vacuum-assisted devices include cephalopelvic disproportion and abnormal presentation. As with forceps delivery, all vacuum-assisted deliveries should be preceded by an assessment of the risks and benefits of cesarean section as an alternative operative option. Episiotomy is not recommended prior to vacuum-assisted delivery due to increased risk of extended perineal laceration.

The steps involved in the use of vacuum assist to effect delivery are as follows:

1. Identify specific indication.
2. Rule out contraindications to vacuum-assisted delivery, including assessment of maternal pelvic adequacy (ischial spine prominence, sacral contour, and suprapubic arch size).
3. Assess risks and benefits of cesarean section as an alternative.
4. Determine fetal head presentation.
5. Determine fetal head station.
6. Prepare for cesarean section in case of failed forceps delivery.
7. Place vacuum-assisted device appropriately.

Contraindications to vacuum-assisted delivery include gestational age <34 weeks, non-cephalic presentation, head not engaged, cephalopelvic disproportion, or known fetal bone or bleeding disorder.

Delivery with a vacuum-assisted device is somewhat different than with forceps. The cup is applied over the sagittal suture approximately 3 cm in front of the posterior fontanelle. Negative pressure (vacuum pressure) is developed, and gentle traction is applied with contractions. Traction should not be applied in the absence of contractions, and no attempt should be made to rotate the position of the fetal head. In general, delivery should be expected within a few (~3) contractions and in no more than 20 min. If the infant has not been delivered, the attempt should be considered failed, and cesarean section should be performed.

Cesarean Section

Cesarean section is the operative delivery of the infant through an abdominal and uterine incision. The placenta and membranes are also delivered transabdominally. The indications for cesarean section include all instances when vaginal delivery is either contraindicated or not feasible. For a complete description of cesarean section, providers should consult a text on operative obstetrics.

Chapter 24
Prolonged Labor

Contents

Background... 183
Complications of Labor... 184
   Prolonged Latent-Phase Labor... 184
History.. 185
Physical Examination... 185
Laboratory/Diagnostic Studies... 185
Management.. 185
   Failure to Dilate/Efface.. 186
History.. 186
Physical Examination... 186
Laboratory/Diagnostic Studies... 187
Management.. 187
   Failure to Descend.. 188

> **Key Points**
> 1. Complications of labor include prolonged transition from latent- to active-phase labor, failure of cervical dilation, and failure to descend.
> 2. Diagnosis of an abnormality of labor requires a firm understanding of the normal progress of labor.
> 3. Each complication of labor requires individual assessment and management.

Background

Most pregnancies will proceed with a minimum of abnormality, and delivery will occur without significant complications. All deliveries have the potential for complications; providers should be aware of and prepared for the potential complications associated with the delivery of the infant.

© Springer Nature Switzerland AG 2020   183
P. Lyons, N. McLaughlin, *Obstetrics in Family Medicine*, Current Clinical Practice,
https://doi.org/10.1007/978-3-030-39888-0_24

Complications of Labor

Labor is defined as uterine contractions resulting in progressive cervical dilation, effacement, and eventual delivery of the infant. The normal course of labor is reviewed in Chap. 19. In general the progression of labor depends on three identifiable factors: adequate uterine contraction (both frequency and force), fetal size and position, and adequate pelvic anatomy to allow descent. Routine labor management includes sequential assessment of labor progress via manual examination of the cervix and presenting fetal body part. Although labor is predictable and progressive in most patients, under some circumstances, the normal progression is disturbed. These may include a delay in the transition from latent- to active-phase labor, failure of cervical dilation to occur, and occurrence of dilation without fetal descent.

Prolonged Latent-Phase Labor

Latent-phase or early labor is the period marked by contractions and initial cervical dilation. The contractions are generally frequent and less strong than those of active labor, and the progress of cervical dilation may be variable. Although average latent-phase labor lasts between 5 and 8 h, there is considerable variability. Often, the management of latent-phase labor occurs outside the medical facility. Ideally, patients without obstetrical complications or medical risk factors would arrive at the hospital in active labor, having self-managed the latent phase of labor.

Under some circumstances, however, patients will present for management while in latent-phase labor. When the latent phase of labor has continued significantly beyond the expected duration, management decisions must be made. The traditional understanding of the latent phase of labor defined "prolonged" latent phase as >20 h for nulliparous women and >14 h for multiparous women. However, more recent review of the data suggests that the latent phase is actually considerably longer and now would be more appropriately understood to be >30 h nulliparous, >24.5 h multiparous. Regardless of how it is defined, most patients with prolonged latent-phase labor will progress to active labor and subsequent vaginal delivery.

Because of the high level of variability and potentially unpredictable course of latent-phase labor, the American College of Obstetricians and Gynecologists recommend that arrest of labor diagnosis be limited to those patients with >6 cm cervical dilation, ruptured membranes, and no cervical change for 4–6 h.

History

Management begins with a review of the patient's history. Review of the gestational age, prenatal course, and prior obstetrical history, if any, should be performed. Although most instances of prolonged latent-phase labor are idiopathic, the use of sedation and alcohol and prior episodes of prolonged labor may all be associated with a prolonged latent phase.

Physical Examination

Assessment of cervical status is the key physical finding. Cervical dilation, effacement, and fetal descent should all be noted. Rupture of membranes should also be noted, as management will vary if membranes are ruptured. Documentation at regular intervals will assist in determining the rate of labor progression and the degree to which the current pregnancy deviates from the norm. As feto–pelvic disproportion may contribute to a prolonged latent-phase assessment of fetal size, presentation and pelvic adequacy should be noted.

Laboratory/Diagnostic Studies

Generally, diagnostic studies are of limited value in the management of prolonged latent-phase labor. Obstetrical ultrasound may assist in assessment of fetal size, and examination of pooled vaginal fluids, if any, may contribute to assessment of possible rupture of membranes. Fetal heart tones should be monitored intermittently to assess fetal well-being.

Management

Most patients with prolonged latent-phase labor require no specific intervention. Of patients with latent-phase labor, 10–15% will show little if any cervical change. These patients have not yet started true labor and may be sent home to rest or walk, with precautions concerning when to return. Rest and hydration will result in active labor in the majority of patients (80–85%) who are kept in the hospital. A small percentage (5–10%) will demonstrate active uterine contractions but insufficient cervical dilation. These patients may benefit from the use of oxytocin to augment labor. Patients with ruptured membranes should be admitted and monitored for signs or symptoms of infection. Details concerning the management of such patients can be found in Chap. 8.

Failure to Dilate/Efface

With the onset of active labor, most patients can be expected to follow a predictable pattern of cervical dilation and effacement. As noted in Chap. 19, expected dilation is approximately 1 cm per hour for primigravid patients and 1.2–1.5 cm per hour for multiparous patients. Total duration of active first-stage labor is approximately 10 h (6–18 h) for primigravid and 5 h (2–10) for multiparous patients. Documented failure to dilate at the expected rate despite the presence of organized uterine contractions is a second complication of labor.

   The underlying etiology for failed cervical dilation is not well understood. Broadly understood, the problem may be with the fetus (size, presentation), with the birth canal (feto–pelvic disproportion), or with the uterine forces necessary to complete expulsion of the fetus. Evaluation of failure to dilate requires assessment of each of these components.

History

The history may contribute to assessment of risk factors associated with either the fetus or the birth canal. The patient's prenatal course should be reviewed, with a particular emphasis on malpresentation and risk factors for macrosomia such as gestational diabetes. Past obstetrical history should also be reviewed for prior failure to dilate, past history of gestational diabetes, or prior macrosomic infants. Feto–pelvic disproportion is largely a diagnosis of exclusion; however, those patients with bony abnormalities of the birth canal can be expected to have recurrent difficulties.

Physical Examination

Physical examination contributes significantly to the diagnosis and management of delayed cervical dilation. Serial cervical examination to assess dilation, effacement, and station should be performed and the results plotted on a normal labor curve. Identification of abnormal presentation may be apparent on physical examination. Abnormal presentations such as occiput posterior, brow, or face presentation occur in approximately 5% of all deliveries and should generally be apparent on examination. Breech presentation with abnormal presentation of fetal body parts may also be determined on pelvic examination. An assessment of fetal size should be performed, as ultrasound assessment of fetal size at term may be inaccurate. Although the reliability of manual assessment of pelvic adequacy has been questioned, a brief evaluation of the birth canal should also be performed as a part of the pelvic examination.

Critical to the assessment and management of prolonged dilation is an assessment of the adequacy of uterine contractions. Although external monitors may be useful for determining the frequency of uterine contractions, determination of the strength of those contractions requires the placement of an intrauterine pressure catheter (IUPC).

Laboratory/Diagnostic Studies

In general, laboratory and diagnostic studies are limited in the management of delayed cervical dilation. An obstetrical ultrasound may assist in the assessment of fetal size or presentation.

Management

Management of delayed cervical dilation requires assessment of which, if any, identifiable factors are contributing to the delay. The management of malpresentation is covered later. The indications for operative delivery are reviewed in Chap. 21.

In the absence of clearly contributory factors such as malpresentation or macrosomia, adequacy of uterine contractions should be assessed. Placement of an IUPC allows for calculation of the adequacy of uterine contractile activity. The most common and simplest measure of uterine activity is the Montevideo unit, measured as the increase in intrauterine pressure with contractions (maximum pressure–baseline pressure) over a 10-min period. The Montevideo units for each contraction are calculated, and all contractions in a 10-min period are added together. A total of 200 Montevideo units are considered evidence of adequate uterine contractile activity.

For patients without adequate uterine contractile activity, oxytocin augmentation should be administered until adequate contractions are established. Cervical dilation should be periodically documented thereafter. Failure to dilate may be diagnosed with 2 h of adequate uterine contractions and no cervical change. If cervical dilation is occurring, management depends on the status of the infant. Slow but steady cervical dilation (with or without oxytocin augmentation) should be allowed to progress unless evidence of fetal stress is noted.

Patients for whom inadequate uterine contractile activity is the only apparent source of incomplete cervical dilation will generally have an excellent outcome, with two-thirds eventually delivering vaginally.

Failure to Descend

Despite full cervical dilation, the fetus may fail to descend through the birth canal. Although inadequate uterine contractile activity contributes to many of these cases, feto–pelvic disproportion makes up roughly half of them. Evaluation is similar to that for failure to dilate. Particular attention should be paid to clinical evidence of pelvic adequacy, fetal size, and malpresentation. If clinical evidence suggests feto–pelvic disproportion, consideration should be given to cesarean section delivery. In the absence of clinical evidence of feto–pelvic disproportion, assessment of uterine activity adequacy and oxytocin augmentation, if necessary, would be indicated.

Chapter 25
Shoulder Dystocia

Contents

Background.. 189
Diagnosis... 190
Management.. 191

> **Key Points**
> 1. Clinically, shoulder dystocia may be diagnosed when delivery of the head is followed by an inability to deliver the shoulders.
> 2. Shoulder dystocia is a serious complication of delivery and must be managed rapidly to minimize maternal and fetal morbidity.

Background

Shoulder dystocia is an uncommon but serious complication of delivery. Clinically, shoulder dystocia may be diagnosed when delivery of the head is followed by an inability to deliver the shoulders. Shoulder dystocia generally requires additional maneuvers to free the shoulders and effect delivery of the infant. Although the exact mechanism is not well studied, the postulated mechanism is impaction of the anterior shoulder against the maternal symphysis pubis or impaction of the posterior shoulder on the sacrum. Rarely, dystocia may be the result of or may be made worse by impaction against the soft tissue of the birth canal.

The risk for shoulder dystocia is approximately 1 in 100 for normal-size infants. A variety of risk factors (*see* Table 25.1) have been associated with an increased risk for dystocia, including prior history of shoulder dystocia, known anatomic abnormalities of the birth canal, gestational diabetes, postdates pregnancy, macrosomia, and protracted labor. Although most cases cannot be identified on the basis

P. Lyons, N. McLaughlin, *Obstetrics in Family Medicine*, Current Clinical Practice,
https://doi.org/10.1007/978-3-030-39888-0_25

Table 25.1 Risk factors for
shoulder dystocia

Assisted delivery
Protracted labor
Postdates pregnancy
Macrosomia
Diabetes
Constitutional short stature
Abnormal pelvic anatomy
Prior shoulder dystocia
Prior macrosomic infant

of identifiable risk factors, infant size is clearly related to an increased risk for dystocia. Macrosomic infants (>4000 g) have a five- to tenfold increase in risk (absolute risk 5–9%).

The complications of shoulder dystocia include direct trauma to the mother and/ or infant, hemorrhage, and, less commonly, possible complications of the delivery itself. Direct trauma to the mother may result in laceration, extension of episiotomy, and postpartum hemorrhage. Approximately 10% of deliveries with shoulder dystocia result in postpartum hemorrhage (for management, *see* Chap. 30). Approximately 3–4% of deliveries will result in fourth-degree lacerations or extensions of an existing episiotomy. Although the connection between birth trauma and subsequent neonatal outcomes is not clear, approximately 10% of all deliveries complicated by shoulder dystocia will result in brachial plexus palsy. Of these, approximately 10% will be persistent. An increased risk for clavicular fracture is also associated with shoulder dystocia.

The management of shoulder dystocia is critical to minimize the medical complications associated with its presentation. Despite appropriate management, shoulder dystocia is associated with an increased risk for clavicular fracture, humeral fracture, fetal hypoxia, and fetal death.

Diagnosis

As noted, shoulder dystocia is a clinical diagnosis made at the time of delivery. No such diagnosis can be made prior to the delivery itself. Prenatal patients should, however, be screened for historic risk factors associated with dystocia, including gestational diabetes, prior macrosomic infant, prior shoulder dystocia, known pelvic anatomic abnormalities, or prior deliveries complicated by feto–pelvic disproportion. Risk factors from the current pregnancy should also be reviewed, including macrosomic infant, gestational diabetes, or risk factors for previously undiagnosed macrosomia, including abnormally large weight gain or abnormally large fundal height.

The diagnosis of shoulder dystocia is made at the time of delivery. Following delivery of the fetal head, the fetal shoulders are delivered via gentle downward traction. With delivery of the anterior shoulder, the posterior shoulder and the remainder of the infant body are delivered via upward movement. When shoulder dystocia occurs, the head is delivered, but delivery of the shoulder is impaired and cannot be achieved with reasonable levels of traction. On occasion, the provider may notice that the head is delivered with a contraction but subsequently retracts with the cessation of the contraction (like a turtle retracting its head back into the shell). When normal traction fails to deliver the shoulders, the diagnosis of dystocia should be made, and management should be immediately instituted.

Management

Patients at risk for shoulder dystocia should be managed from the onset of labor with the anticipation that shoulder dystocia will occur. All delivery room personnel should be aware of the risk, all necessary equipment should be available in the room, and delivery should be performed with sufficient support staff available to immediately begin management if necessary. In addition, some experts recommend immediate delivery of the anterior shoulder with the head for patients who are at high risk for shoulder dystocia. This maneuver, although widely recommended, has not been well studied in clinical trials.

With the diagnosis of shoulder dystocia, management should begin immediately, as outlined in Table 25.2. Each intervention is completed in a stepwise manner until the infant is delivered:

1. If sufficient assistance is not available in the room, help should be summoned immediately, and staff should be made aware of the situation.
2. Following failure of gentle traction to deliver the shoulders, the patient should be positioned with hips flexed and abducted (McRoberts maneuver), and suprapubic pressure should be applied while the patient pushes. It should be noted that fundal pressure is contraindicated; pressure should be downward and administered just above the symphysis pubis.
3. If delivery is not achieved with these maneuvers, an episiotomy may be performed to decrease soft tissue dystocia and facilitate delivery.

Table 25.2 Management of shoulder dystocia

Get assistance
Flex and abduct hips
Suprapubic pressure (*not* fundal pressure)
Shoulder rotation
Anterior shoulder forward
Posterior shoulder backward
Posterior shoulder forward
Reposition patient on all fours
Emergency maneuvers

4. If delivery is still not achieved, internal rotation of the infant's shoulders should be attempted. The anterior shoulder is rotated forward (pressure is applied from behind the anterior shoulder directed forward from the infant's perspective). This is followed by rotating the posterior shoulder backward (pressure on the anterior surface, the shoulder should be directed backward from the infant's perspective). This is performed while maintaining the forward pressure on the anterior shoulder.
5. If delivery has not been achieved, then forward rotation of the posterior shoulder is attempted followed by delivery of the posterior arm/shoulder. The posterior arm is swept forward across the infant's chest and elbow flexed.
6. Repositioning the patient on all fours may sufficiently alter the position and forces to allow for delivery of the infant.
7. If all of the above have failed to deliver the infant, immediate emergency maneuvers will be required to effect delivery. These may include clavicular fracture and/or replacing the head in the birth canal followed by cesarean section (Zavanelli maneuver).

Chapter 26
Malpresentation

Contents

Background... 193
Occiput Positions.. 194
   Diagnosis.. 194
   Management... 194
Nonoccipital Presentations.. 194
Breech Presentation.. 195
Compound Presentation... 196

Key Points

1. Normal delivery is marked by a characteristic fetal presentation and a stereotyped series of fetal repositions.
2. Failure to present in the usual occiput anterior position may lead to prolongation and complications of labor and may be incompatible with vaginal delivery.
3. Careful assessment of fetal presentation is critical to the diagnosis and management of abnormal presentations.

Background

Although fetal position during the prenatal period is variable and subject to change (especially prior to 36 weeks' gestation), most infants will arrive head first and neck flexed with the occiput (either right or left occiput) in an anterior position. Variations from this position and presentation do occur, however, and providers should be aware of possible variants. Assessment of fetal presentation should be a routine component of late prenatal care and with all patients at the time of labor. Complications with the progress of labor, as noted earlier, should prompt reevaluation of fetal presentation and position.

© Springer Nature Switzerland AG 2020 193
P. Lyons, N. McLaughlin, *Obstetrics in Family Medicine*, Current Clinical Practice,
https://doi.org/10.1007/978-3-030-39888-0_26

Occiput Positions

Occipital position is described in relation to the anterior surface of the mother. In the usual dorsal lithotomy position, this will place the anterior surface upward. In the normal presentation, the fetus will present vertex first with the occipital portion of the skull in an anterior location (occiput anterior, occiput toward the symphysis pubis, upward in the usual dorsal lithotomy position). The occiput may, however, be either posterior (occiput away from the symphysis or downward in the dorsal lithotomy position) or transverse (occiput horizontal or to the side in the dorsal lithotomy position). With the onset of labor, most infants will already be in the occiput anterior position. Approximately 20%, however, will be positioned in an alternative position at the beginning of labor. For most of these infants, occiput posterior or occiput transverse is only a temporary position that will revert to occiput anterior during the course of delivery. Fewer than 5% of infants will present with occiput posterior or occiput transverse at the time of delivery.

Diagnosis

Diagnosis of fetal position is made via manual examination at the time of delivery. Examination should reveal anterior and posterior fontanelles as well as the normal fetal suture lines. These three landmarks should be sufficient to determine the orientation of the fetal head.

Management

Occiput posterior and occiput transverse positions are both compatible with vaginal delivery although their presence is associated with a higher rate of assisted or surgical deliveries. If fetal size is within normal limits and there is no evidence of pelvic abnormalities, rotation of the fetal head may be considered. The use of forceps should be limited to patients without the above abnormalities and should only be performed by a provider with considerable experience with the use of forceps. In the absence of such an experienced provider, in the presence of macrosomia, feto–pelvic disproportion, or with prolonged failure of dilation or descent, cesarean delivery may be indicated.

Nonoccipital Presentations

Although occipital (or vertex) presentation is the most common presentation, other presentations are possible. Brow presentations (partially deflexed neck) are uncommon and are generally self-limited. Approximately 50% of such presentations will revert to vertex presentation with the continuation of labor. Brow presentation at the time of delivery occurs less than 1 in 1000 births. Diagnosis is made by manual examination, and management consists of continued management with an expectation of vaginal delivery. If the patient has been on oxytocin, this should be discontinued to minimize the possibility of dystocia. Failure of brow presentation to revert to vertex presentation is associated with a high likelihood of dystocia and is an indication for cesarean delivery. Face presentations represent fully deflexed neck position with the face descending the birth canal in the lead position. Face presentation is more common than a brow presentation but is still uncommon, only occurring approximately 2 per 1000 deliveries. The retroflexion of the fetal neck combined with the presentation of the chin as the presenting body part significantly increases the likelihood of cephalopelvic disproportion and is not generally compatible with vaginal delivery. If the chin is in a posterior position (mentum posterior), cesarean delivery is indicated. If the chin is in an anterior position, vaginal delivery may be attempted, but such an attempt carries a higher-than-expected risk of failure and subsequent cesarean delivery.

Breech Presentation

Although most infants will descend the birth canal in a head-first position, a small number will present with an alternative presenting part. Such abnormal positions can be determined during prenatal care and as such should be noted at all visits in the last 2 months of the prenatal course. Breech presentation at term but prior to labor may be amenable to manipulation/rotation (external cephalic version) to position the infant's head in a downward position. External version should be done at approximately 37 weeks' gestation to minimize the likelihood of reversion and should be done in a setting that allows for management of labor, including tocolysis. External version is an indication for the use of rhogam in Rh-negative patients. Between one- and two-thirds of such procedures are successful (defined as vertex presentation at the onset of labor).

Breech presentations may be classified by the presenting body part and the position of the fetal body. Frank breech implies buttock presentation with flexion at the hips and extension of the knees (in essence, folded in half at the hips with the buttock in the birth canal and the head at the uterine fundus). Complete breech is buttock presentation with both hips and knees flexed (the typical "fetal position" with buttock presentation and the head near the uterine fundus). An incomplete breech— sometimes referred to as a footling breech—implies presentation of one or more of the lower extremities. In the United States, delivery of breech presentation is generally via cesarean section, although optimal management remains controversial. If vaginal delivery is to be attempted, all of the following should be true: at or near term in labor with no evidence of fetal stress, frank breech presentation with full neck flexion, normal fetal size (2500–3800 g), no known congenital abnormalities, and no known pelvic abnormalities. Only providers with experience in the use of piper forceps and with cesarean backup ready at the time of delivery should perform such an attempt.

Compound Presentation

Compound presentation is the presentation of an arm or leg along with the presenting part. It is most commonly associated with either small infants or large birth
canals. The most common variant is presentation of a hand along with the head.
Diagnosis is made on manual examination at the time of labor, and management
generally consists of expectant vaginal delivery. Care should be exercised to determine that the umbilical cord has not prolapsed along with the compound body part.
In addition, providers should be prepared to proceed to cesarean section in the case
of fetal compromise, failure of dilation or descent, or dystocia. Repositioning of the
presenting body part is generally not recommended.

Chapter 27
Fetal Heart Rate Monitoring

Contents

Background.. 197
  Normal Fetal Heart Tracings.. 198
Evaluation of Fetal Heart Rate Baseline... 198
  Tachycardia... 199
  Bradycardia... 199
Evaluation of Fetal Heart Rate Variability.. 199
  Acceleration.. 199
  Early Deceleration.. 200
  Variable Deceleration.. 200
  Late Decelerations.. 200
Classification of Electronic Fetal Monitoring... 201

Key Points

1. The common use of continuous fetal heart rate monitoring requires that providers be aware of the interpretation of variations in fetal heart tracings.
2. Normal fetal heart rate is 110–160 beats per minute (bpm) with evidence of short- and long-term variability.
3. Fetal heart rate acceleration must be distinguished from fetal tachycardia and is generally considered a favorable finding.
4. Abnormalities of fetal heart tracings may be related to either rate or deceleration.

Background

The advent of electronic fetal heart rate monitoring has dramatically changed intra-partum management within the United States. The almost universal presence of such monitoring during the course of most deliveries presents providers with a variety of

© Springer Nature Switzerland AG 2020

P. Lyons, N. McLaughlin, *Obstetrics in Family Medicine*, Current Clinical Practice,
https://doi.org/10.1007/978-3-030-39888-0_27

challenges. Controversy exists concerning the clinical benefit of continuous electronic fetal monitoring. Such controversy, however, does not eliminate the need for obstetrical providers to be familiar with the basics of electronic fetal monitoring, normal and abnormal findings, and appropriate management for abnormal tracings.

Normal Fetal Heart Tracings

Routine fetal heart tracing should be evaluated for baseline heart rate as well as variation from that baseline rate. Normal baseline fetal heart rate during pregnancy is between 110 and 160 bpm. The baseline heart rate may be determined by examining a fetal heart tracing of sufficient length to determine the heart rate to which the tracing consistently returns. It may be helpful to use a ruler or other straight edge along the course of a fetal heart rate tracing to help determine the baseline value. Fetal heart rate tracing should demonstrate a degree of variability over the course of time. A fetal heart rate tracing with little evidence of variability requires careful monitoring and evaluation if persistent.

Once the baseline fetal heart rate has been determined, variation from this baseline should also be noted. Is should be apparent that this variation from baseline may be in either direction. Variation upward (toward higher fetal heart rate) is referred to as *acceleration*, whereas variation downward (toward lower fetal heart rates) is referred to as *deceleration*. In addition to the absolute direction of movement, a note should be made of patterns of fetal heart rate activity that may be indicative of careful follow-up or intervention. Nonreassuring fetal heart rate patterns are outlined in Table 27.1.

Evaluation of Fetal Heart Rate Baseline

The baseline fetal heart rate may, under some circumstances, vary from the normal range of 110–160 bpm. When the baseline is determined to vary from this normal range, a careful review of potential causes should be performed.

Table 27.1 Nonreassuring fetal heart rate patterns

Fetal tachycardia (persistently >160 bpm)
Fetal bradycardia (persistently <110 bpm)
Variable deceleration (decelerations with onset mid-contraction)
Late deceleration with or without short-term variability (decelerations with onset after peak of contraction)
Prolonged severe bradycardia (persistently or recurrently <100 bpm)
Sinusoidal pattern (smooth, rounded, wavelike pattern)

bpm beats per minute

Tachycardia

Tachycardia is defined as a baseline at or above 160 bpm. Mild tachycardia is defined as 160–180 bpm. Severe tachycardia is defined as more than 180 bpm. Fetal tachycardia may be associated with fetal hypoxia, maternal fever, drug or medication use, infection, fetal cardiac abnormalities, anemia, and hyperthyroidism. Persistent tachycardia should prompt review of potential causes and intervention if indicated.

Bradycardia

Fetal bradycardia is defined as a baseline at or below 110 bpm. A variety of conditions may produce bradycardia in the range of 100–110 bpm. If variability is good and no other abnormalities are noted, careful monitoring may be sufficient. Prolonged or severe fetal bradycardia may be associated with cord compression or prolapse, anesthesia, uterine tetany, or rapid descent of the fetus through the birth canal.

Evaluation of Fetal Heart Rate Variability

Once the baseline fetal heart rate has been determined, variation from this baseline should also be noted. This variation from baseline may be in either direction. Variation upward (toward higher fetal heart rate) is referred to as *acceleration*, whereas variation downward (toward lower fetal heart rates) is referred to as *deceleration*. In addition to the absolute direction of movement, note should be made of patterns of fetal heart rate activity that may be indicative of careful follow-up or intervention.

Acceleration

In contrast to a persistent rise in baseline fetal heart rate (tachycardia), fetal heart rate acceleration is generally a favorable finding and may be associated with fetal stimulation (e.g., with contractions or cervical examinations). Fetal heart rate acceleration following variable deceleration (*see* below) is a common finding and is generally considered a good prognostic indicator.

Early Deceleration

Early decelerations are defined by a slow onset that coincides with the onset of contractions. The decelerations are thought to correspond to fetal head compression and are considered reassuring. The slow onset is matched by a similarly slow recovery producing a symmetric shape that corresponds with the duration of the contraction.

Variable Deceleration

As implied by its name, the onset, shape, and recovery of variable decelerations is less uniform than for either early or late decelerations. Interpretation of variable deceleration is likewise dependent on the associated clinical factors and the specific findings noted on the tracing. In general, variable decelerations have a relatively rapid onset and recovery with a shape that resembles a "V." As noted earlier, variable decelerations are often associated with accelerations immediately preceding onset and immediately following recovery, yielding a pattern that resembles shoulders. Variable decelerations are thought to be associated with umbilical cord compression and their interpretation is therefore dependent of the potential causes of such compression. Mild decelerations are of less than 30 s in duration and are no lower than 80 bpm at their nadir. Moderate decelerations last between 30 and 60 s and reach 70–80 bpm at the nadir. Severe variable contractions last longer than 1 min and/or reach less than 70 bpm at the nadir. Several findings on the tracing are considered nonreassuring in the assessment of variable decelerations. These include increasing frequency or severity, delayed recovery, decreased variability, and loss of associated accelerations ("shoulders").

Late Decelerations

Late decelerations are characterized by an onset at or after the peak of the associated uterine contraction. Distinguishing late decelerations from persistent variable decelerations may be difficult under some circumstances. Late decelerations are thought to be related to uteroplacental insufficiency and are often indicative of fetal hypoxia. Conditions associated with an increased risk for late decelerations include diabetes, hypertension/pre-eclampsia, and postdates pregnancy.

Classification of Electronic Fetal Monitoring

All tracings should fall into one of three categories:

- *Category 1*—tracing shows a normal baseline with moderate variability and not variable or late decelerations. A Category 1 tracing may or may not demonstrate accelerations.
- *Category 2*—tracing that does not fall into either category 1 or category 3.
- *Category 3*—tracing demonstrates limited or absent variability with recurrent variable decelerations, recurrent late decelerations, persistent bradycardia, or a persistent sinusoidal pattern.

Chapter 28
Maternal Fever in Labor

Contents

Background... 203
Diagnosis... 204
   History... 204
   Physical Examination... 204
   Diagnostic Studies... 205
Management... 205

> **Key Points**
> 1. Labor may be complicated by maternal infection with associated maternal and neonatal risk.
> 2. Management of maternal fever requires a knowledge of the common sources of infection and appropriate antibiotic coverage for those organisms.
> 3. Management of maternal infection requires an awareness of the risks and benefits of antibiotic use in pregnancy.

Background

Maternal fever ($T \geq 38$ °C, 100.4 °F) during the course of labor is surprisingly uncommon given the number of potential pathogens in the genitourinary (GU) and gastrointestinal (GI) tracts and the nonsterile conditions of labor and delivery. Despite the relative rarity of maternal fever, providers should monitor maternal temperature regularly and be prepared to intervene appropriately if maternal fever develops. In general intraamniotic infection should be presumed in patients with fever. Isolated maternal fever is defined as a maternal temperature >38.0 and <39.0 with no additional risk factors noted. Any measured temperature at or above 39.0

© Springer Nature Switzerland AG 2020
P. Lyons, N. McLaughlin, *Obstetrics in Family Medicine*, Current Clinical Practice,
https://doi.org/10.1007/978-3-030-39888-0_28

Table 28.1 Diagnosis of intraamniotic infection

Temperature (persistent over 30 min or more)	Associated symptoms/risk factors	Diagnosis
38.0–38.9	Absent	Isolated maternal fever
38.0–38.9	Present	Suspected intraamniotic infection
39.0+	Absent	Suspected intraamniotic infection
39.0+	Present	Confirmed intraamniotic infection

with or without additional risk factors should be considered diagnostic of chorioamnionitis (this is summarized in Table 28.1). Maternal risk factors include persistent elevated fetal heart rate, elevated maternal white blood cell count, or purulent cervical discharge.

Diagnosis

History

The prenatal history should be reviewed for prior infection as well as risk factors for intrapartum infection. In particular, the results from any recent testing for gonorrhea, chlamydia, group B streptococcus, urinary tract infection, and bacterial vaginosis should be noted. Although herpes and syphilis infections are not usually associated with fever, both should be noted if present. Prior antibiotic use should be documented.

The nature and timing of rupture of membranes should also be noted. In addition, manipulation should be reviewed including artificial rupture of membranes, frequent manual cervical checks, or placement of fetal scalp electrodes, intrauterine pressure catheters, or bladder catheter placement.

Although less common, respiratory sources should be considered in laboring patients with fever. History should also include a review of the patients' PHx and exposures prior to labor to identify additional possible etiologies.

Physical Examination

Physical examination should include documentation of maternal temperature, blood pressure, and pulse. Maternal fever may be associated with fetal tachycardia; therefore, fetal heart rate should also be documented. Examination of the lungs for abnormal lung sounds should be performed. Abdominal examination may reveal abdominal tenderness. Although vaginal discharge may be difficult to determine during labor, sterile pelvic examination may also be indicated.

Diagnostic Studies

Although not all maternal fevers are infectious, all such fevers should be assumed to be of infectious etiology until proven otherwise. Blood and urine cultures should be sent. If not previously performed, gonorrhea, chlamydia, and group B streptococcus testing should performed. A complete blood count should be reviewed. Although the maternal white blood cell count may be elevated in pregnancy, an elevated white blood cell count in the setting of maternal fever is one of three identified associated symptoms indicative of suspected intraamniotic infection.

Management

As noted, fever should be assumed to be infectious until proven otherwise. Administration of appropriate antibiotic therapy may be of benefit to both the mother and the fetus. Specifically, the use of antibiotics in suspected or confirmed chorioamnionitis is associated with decreased risk of neonatal sepsis, and decreased maternal length of stay. If a specific etiology is known, antibiotic choice should be dictated by the sensitivity of that infectious agent. If no specific etiology is noted, broad-spectrum antibiotic coverage sufficient to cover routine GU and GI flora should be initiated. Antibiotic regimens that meet these criteria include:

1. Ampicillin and gentamicin
2. Cefazolin and gentamicin
3. Clindamycin or vancomycin and gentamicin (if penicillin allergic)

Maternal fever in labor should prompt early and thorough evaluation of the infant following delivery. There is controversy regarding the use of antibiotics for infants born to mothers with chorioamnionitis. Most guidelines currently recommend universal antibiotics. With or without antibiotics, close clinical surveillance is critical.

Chapter 29
Postpartum Hemorrhage

Contents

Background.. 208
Complications Causing Hemorrhage.. 208
  Uterine Atony... 208
  Lacerations... 209
  Retained Placenta.. 209
  Coagulopathy.. 209
  Uterine Inversion... 209
Diagnosis... 209
Management.. 210
  Laceration.. 210
  Persistent Bleeding.. 211

> **Key Points**
> 1. Postpartum hemorrhage may result from lacerations, retained placenta, uterine inversion, or coagulopathy.
> 2. Management of postpartum hemorrhage begins prior to delivery with assessment of precedent risk factors including macrosomia, polyhydramnios, precipitous labor, grand multiparity, anesthesia, augmentation, and caesarian delivery. Active management of the third stage of labor is associated with decreased risk of postpartum hemorrhage.
> 3. Postpartum hemorrhage is a critical postpartum complication that requires rapid identification and management.
> 4. Management of postpartum hemorrhage should proceed in a stepwise manner until hemorrhage is controlled.

© Springer Nature Switzerland AG 2020
P. Lyons, N. McLaughlin, *Obstetrics in Family Medicine*, Current Clinical Practice,
https://doi.org/10.1007/978-3-030-39888-0_29

Background

Postpartum hemorrhage complicates approximately 5% of all deliveries. It is the second leading cause of maternal mortality in the United States, causing approximately 12% of all such deaths. All deliveries are associated with blood loss. Postpartum hemorrhage is defined as blood loss of at least 1000 cc or blood loss associated with symptoms of hypovolemia. Actual blood loss during the course of routine delivery may exceed 500 cc if carefully measured. Although the definition of postpartum hemorrhage remains unchanged, from a practical standpoint, postpartum hemorrhage is often understood as hemorrhage that persists beyond expectation. Early (primary) postpartum hemorrhage is defined as blood loss occurring in the first 24 h postpartum. Late (secondary) postpartum hemorrhage is defined as blood loss occurring between 24 h and 12 weeks' postpartum.

Following delivery of the infant, normal bleeding is controlled by separation of the placenta, uterine contraction with constriction of placental bed vessels, and normal hemostatic pathways. Postpartum hemorrhage occurs when one or more of these events are disrupted. Postpartum hemorrhage may be caused by a variety of obstetrical complications including uterine atony, lacerations, retained placenta, and obstetrically related coagulopathy. Most cases of postpartum hemorrhage are caused by obstetrical complications; however, providers should also be aware that pre-existing coagulopathies may also manifest as postpartum hemorrhage.

Complications Causing Hemorrhage

Uterine Atony

Following routine delivery, myometrial contraction results in vascular constriction and control of bleeding. A variety of conditions may result in diminished myometrial contraction and subsequent uterine atony. Factors associated with an increased risk of uterine atony include (a) anatomic conditions such as leiomyosis; (b) uterine distention from such conditions as multigestation, polyhydramnios, or macrosomia; (c) labor-related factors such as prolonged or precipitous delivery; (d) management factors such as anesthesia, augmentation/induction, or caesarian delivery; (e) maternal factors such as multiparity; and (f) postpartum complications such as infection. Uterine atony is responsible for 50% of postpartum hemorrhage cases.

Lacerations

Delivery often results in trauma to the birth canal and may result in lacerations to the uterus, cervix, vagina, or perineum. Significant lacerations are associated with both precipitous and operative delivery. Although bleeding from such lacerations is generally self-limited or controlled with routine repair, lacerations are responsible for up to 20% of postpartum hemorrhage cases.

Retained Placenta

Retained placenta represents the third significant cause of postpartum hemorrhage. Approximately 10% of cases are related to this cause.

Coagulopathy

Although relatively uncommon, a number of obstetrical complications may lead to coagulopathy, which may in turn lead to persistent postpartum bleeding. Factors associated with coagulopathy include fetal demise, amniotic fluid embolus, pre-eclampsia/eclampsia, sepsis, and abruptio placenta.

Uterine Inversion

Under some circumstances, the uterine fundus may invert, preventing myometrial contraction and vascular constriction.

Diagnosis

Diagnosis is generally straightforward and consists of persistent bleeding that exceeds expected levels following delivery. Although the exact blood loss may be difficult to quantify, any suspicion of excess blood loss should lead to an immediate investigation of potential causes. In addition, providers should have a low index of suspicion for initiating general management steps, as postpartum hemorrhage may be both rapid and severe.

Management

Management of postpartum hemorrhage begins prior to delivery. Patients with pre-disposing risk factors should be identified and complications should be anticipated. For patients with significant predisposing risk factors, intravenous access and cross-matched blood products should be arranged prior to delivery. Patients for whom blood product transfusions would be declined should be identified prior to delivery.

The risk of postpartum hemorrhage may also be reduced with appropriate management of delivery. The delivery should be controlled, operative deliveries should be minimized, routine use of episiotomy should be avoided, and active management of the third stage of labor should be routinely employed.

Active management of the third stage of labor consists of three related but distinct steps. The first step is administration of oxytocin with the delivery of the anterior shoulder. Following delivery of the infant, sustained gentle cord traction (Brandt-Andrews maneuver) should be maintained. Finally, with delivery of the placenta, uterine massage should be employed.

Despite appropriate predelivery and postpartum management, postpartum hemorrhage may occur. Because postpartum hemorrhage may represent a life-threatening complication, initial steps should be taken to ensure hemodynamic stability. Blood should be typed and crossmatched. Intravenous access should be established preferably with two large-bore access sites. Patient blood pressure should be closely monitored. Significant drops in blood pressure should lead to initiation of fluid support with either intravenous fluid or blood products. In addition, appropriate labs should be sent including a complete blood count and a coagulation panel.

While performing the measures mentioned above, a review of risk factors should be performed and common causes explored. Uterine tone should be assessed. A comprehensive inspection of the perineum, vagina, and cervix should be performed. Under some circumstances, exploration of the uterine cavity (either manually or via ultrasound) may also be indicated.

Laceration

Significant lacerations will require repair. The presence of laceration does not preclude the possibility of either uterine atony or coagulopathy. Repair of lacerations does not necessarily ensure the cessation of bleeding, and such bleeding must be managed as noted here if it persists.

Persistent Bleeding

Management of persistent bleeding will generally follow a stepwise approach:

1. Uterine massage: fundal massage of the uterus will often result in myometrial contraction and control of the bleeding. It should be noted that massage may need to be repeated. Alternately bimanual uterine massage (one hand in the vagina, one at the fundus) may also be effective. Simultaneous with massage, IV access should be obtained if not already done, oxygenation should be assessed, and consideration should be given to sending labs to assess coagulation and blood count status as well as type and crossmatch for possible transfusion.
2. Oxytocin should be started with the delivery of the anterior shoulder. Oxytocin may be administered as either 10 U intramuscularly or 40 U in 1 L of normal saline delivered intravenously.
3. For patients with identified postpartum hemorrhage, oxytocin is recommended as first line treatment regardless of prior use for induction, augmentation or active third stage management. Treatment dose is 20–40 U oxytocin in 1 L normal saline, 500 cc bolus followed by 250 cc/hr.
4. Methylergonovine efficacy is similar to oxytocin but is associated with more significant side effects, including a significant rise in blood pressure. The usual dose is 0.2 mg intramuscular. This may be repeated after 2–4 h if necessary.
5. Carboprost (15-methyl-PGF2 alpha): 250 µg IM every 15–90 min with a maximum 2 mg dose.
6. Misoprostil may be used as a primary agent if oxytocin is not available or as a secondary agent. A single sublingual or rectal dose of 400–800 µg is recommended.
7. Tranexamic acid (1 g IV over 10 min) when given within 3 hours of onset of bleeding is associated with reduced mortality secondary to bleeding but is not associated with a reduction in overall mortality.

If bleeding persists despite the measures just given, immediate evaluation for possible surgical or embolization intervention is indicated.

Chapter 30
Perineal Laceration and Episiotomy

Contents

Episiotomy.. 213
   Background... 213
Procedure... 214
Perineal Laceration.. 214
   Background... 214
Diagnosis.. 214
   History... 214
Physical Examination.. 215
Management.. 215

> **Key Points**
> 1. Laceration and episiotomy are common complications of the delivery process.
> 2. Lacerations and extension of episiotomies may be minimized with careful management of delivery.
> 3. Laceration and episiotomy repair is an essential skill for all providers who deliver babies.

Episiotomy

Background

Episiotomy is a planned incision of the perineum designed to facilitate delivery of the infant. Although routine episiotomy is not generally considered indicated, a variety of conditions may require episiotomy. Such conditions include shoulder dystocia, assisted delivery, or an anticipated macrosomic infant. Studies concerning

© Springer Nature Switzerland AG 2020
P. Lyons, N. McLaughlin, *Obstetrics in Family Medicine*, Current Clinical Practice,
https://doi.org/10.1007/978-3-030-39888-0_30

the use of episiotomies to reduce the likelihood of laceration extension to third or fourth degree have shown conflicting results. The roles of episiotomies under the conditions just described, however, have generally been recognized to assist with delivery of the infant.

Procedure

Following appropriate anesthesia (epidural anesthesia if present or local anesthesia if not), preparation is made for surgical incision of the perineum. With early crowning, a sharp incision is made through the perineal tissue. Median episiotomies are directed posterior toward the rectum with caution to avoid the anal sphincter and rectum. Mediolateral episiotomies are directed posteriorly approximately 45° left or right of midline.

Perineal Laceration

Background

Either with or without a planned episiotomy, delivery of an infant may result in laceration of the vagina, perineum, or rectum. Lacerations may involve the vagina, perineum, cervix, or uterus, as well as the vestibular tissue. Careful inspection of each of these areas should occur when postpartum hemorrhage persists beyond the expected interval. Perineal lacerations are graded (first to fourth degree) based on the degree of tissue involvement and the repair varies by laceration type. Generally, an episiotomy is equivalent to a second-degree laceration, but clinical conditions may require a more extensive episiotomy or secondary extension of the episiotomy may increase the degree of involvement. Repair of lacerations and episiotomies are generally similar and are summarized in Table 30.1.

Diagnosis

History

Any delivery may result in laceration; however, some deliveries may increase the risk of laceration. Rapid deliveries, especially those for which control of the exiting head or shoulders could not be maintained, increase the risk. Assisted deliveries (with either forceps or vacuum-assisted devices) are often associated with laceration, are often accompanied by a planned episiotomy, and may also result in a lacerated extension of the episiotomy. Larger infants may increase the risk of laceration.

Table 30.1 Grading of vaginal/perineal lacerations

Degree	Description	Repair
First degree	Superficial laceration involving the skin (vaginal or perineal). These may also be superficial periurethral laceration	Generally no repair is necessary unless persistent bleeding from the site is noted
Second degree	Deeper laceration involving perineal tissue up to but not including the capsule of the anal sphincter	Approximation of laceration tissue with suture repair of laceration
Third degree	Laceration involving the anal sphincter but sparing the rectal mucosa	Approximation and suturing of lacerated ends of the anal sphincter followed by repair of the more superficial tissue as with second-degree laceration
Fourth degree	Laceration involving the rectal mucosa	Repair of the rectal mucosa followed by repair of the sphincter and more superficial tissue as noted above

Deliveries complicated by shoulder dystocia are at increased risk for episiotomy and/or laceration. Prior cesarean section increases the risk of uterine rupture/laceration.

Physical Examination

All deliveries should be followed by thorough inspection of the outlet tract to identify any possible lacerations. Such lacerations may be present in the vagina, the perineum surrounding vestibular tissue, the cervix, or the uterus itself. Careful inspection with appropriate visualization (including retraction when necessary and appropriate lighting) will allow for determination of the presence and degree of lacerations, if any. All identified lacerations should be fully inspected to determine the full extent of tissue damage. This includes both the depth of involvement and the length of the laceration.

Management

Management of a laceration depends on the location and degree of tissue involvement. General principles of management are included in Table 30.1.

First-Degree Lacerations First-degree lacerations will rarely require repair. Careful inspection should be performed to determine that persistent bleeding does not occur at the site, however.

Second-Degree Lacerations Second-degree lacerations will often require repair. Once the extent of the laceration is determined, the area is infiltrated with local anesthesia such as 1% plain lidocaine. Anatomic approximation of the lacerated tissue is critical, although exact approximation may be difficult owing to uneven, irregular, or damaged tissue margins. Repair is usually performed with medium-weight absorbable suture. Repair begins above the apex of the laceration and proceeds toward the vaginal opening to the hymenal ring. Deep tissue of the perineum between the hymenal ring and the rectum is then approximated, followed by repair of the superficial tissue and skin.

Third-Degree Lacerations These lacerations will require repair in almost all cases. The first step involves identification of the lacerated ends of the anal sphincter. Once the ends are secured, repair of the anal sphincter and capsule is performed. The remainder of the repair is similar to that of a second-degree laceration.

Fourth-Degree Lacerations Fourth-degree lacerations are the most significant of the perineal lacerations, with the highest likelihood of both short- and long-term complications. For this reason, repair of fourth-degree lacerations should only be performed by providers with considerable experience and expertise. Consultation with an experienced provider is recommended if personal experience is limited. Repair begins with repair of the rectal laceration, proceeds to repair of the anal sphincter, and is completed with the repair described for second-degree lacerations.

Part V
Postpartum Management

Chapter 31
Newborn Evaluation

Contents

Background.. 220
The Examination.. 220
   History.. 220
   Physical Examination... 220
Vital Signs.. 220
General Observation.. 221
Head and Neck.. 221
Eyes.. 221
Cardiovascular.. 221
Pulmonary/Thoracic... 222
Abdomen.. 222
Genital Examination.. 222
Anus.. 222
Spine... 222
Skin.. 223
Extremities... 223
Neurologic.. 223
   Laboratory and Diagnostic Studies.. 223
   Vaccination... 224

Key Points

1. The newborn examination forms the basis for all subsequent management. It is therefore comprehensive in nature.
2. The newborn evaluation includes a review of prenatal and peripartum history, as well as newborn nursery course and physical examination.

© Springer Nature Switzerland AG 2020
P. Lyons, N. McLaughlin, *Obstetrics in Family Medicine*, Current Clinical Practice,
https://doi.org/10.1007/978-3-030-39888-0_31

Background

The initial newborn examination occurs immediately postpartum and will be repeated each day of the newborn's hospital stay. This examination forms the basis for all subsequent management by providing an assessment of development and congenital abnormalities, if any. This examination is therefore comprehensive in nature.

The Examination

History

The newborn history consists primarily of a review of the prenatal and delivery course, including complications, if any. Particular attention should be made of the family history of congenital abnormalities, maternal medical conditions, and prenatal exposures including infection, medications, tobacco, alcohol, and illicit drugs.

Physical Examination

As noted, the newborn physical examination serves as the baseline comparator for all subsequent examinations. It should, therefore, be comprehensive, detailed, and guided by an understanding of the most common areas of abnormality.

Vital Signs

Vital signs include temperature, pulse, respiratory rate, length, weight, and head circumference. Temperature can be checked in a variety of locations, and the specific location should be noted along with the reading. Pulse and respiratory rate are both measured most accurately with the infant resting quietly, preferably in a parent's arms or lap. Length is often most easily measured by marking the disposable paper on the exam table. A mark can be made at the crown of the head. The infant's legs can be fully extended and a mark is made at his or her heel. The infant is then removed and the distance between the two marks is recorded. The additional weight of clothing and diapers can be significant for infants, so weight should be measured with the infant fully disrobed. Head circumference is measured as the circumference from the brow (above the eyebrows) to the temple (above the ears) and around the occiput (roughly equivalent to the position of a hat band).

General Observation

General observations should include whether the child appears healthy, comfortable, and normal. Skin is generally pink and warm to the touch. The scalp may show evidence of the delivery including small lacerations from the scalp electrode or cephalohematoma. Infants generally rest with arms and legs flexed. Newborns will often cry with the movement of the examination and/or stimulation.

Head and Neck

The face should be observed for rashes. The ear canals should be checked for patency and the ears for position. Also, the preauricular pits should be noted when present. One should check the mouth and soft palate for defects and make note of the mucosal lining for both moisture and oral thrush, if present. Both anterior and posterior fontanelles should be open (soft to touch). The anterior fontanelle is rectangular and larger. The posterior fontanelle is smaller and triangular. The neck should be palpated for adenopathy. When the child is gently raised from the table, the head lag should be noted.

Eyes

All infants should be checked for red reflex and for normal eye movement in all directions. Reaction of pupils to light should be noted. Space between the eyes should be noted as both increased and decreased distance between eyes may be associated with genetic disorders.

Cardiovascular

Although it is often difficult for students to distinguish heart sounds in a rapid infant cardiac cycle, note should be made of S1 and S2 in all infants and murmurs, if present. Congenital heart defects may not be apparent at birth and may be picked up for the first time in the physician's office. Palpate peripheral pulses with particular note made of femoral pulses (both quality and symmetry).

Pulmonary/Thoracic

Normal breath sounds and, if present, adventitial (rales, rhonchi, wheezes) sounds should be noted. Note should be made of the chest wall contour, especially at the sternum; the clavicle should be palpated for uneven contour, which may indicate a fracture. The provider should examine the breasts and palpate for breast tissue.

Abdomen

Particular note should be made of the umbilical stump if present. This generally detaches by 2–4 weeks of age. The umbilical region should also be examined for umbilical hernia, noted as either a palpable defect below the umbilicus or as a visible bulging of the area below the umbilical stump. More significant findings might include gastroschisis, omphalocele (both surgical emergencies), or scaphoid abdomen potentially indicating a diaphragmatic hernia. Palpation is generally unremarkable but may reveal masses. Most such masses arise from the kidneys.

Genital Examination

Males should be examined for the presence of both testicles. When applicable, the site of circumcision should be inspected. In uncircumcised males, the foreskin should be retracted to examine the glans. In females, patency of the vagina should be noted. The inguinal region should be examined for the presence of congenital hernias.

Anus

The anus should be checked for patency, and note should be made of rashes that might represent either diaper contact dermatitis or candidiasis.

Spine

The entire course of the spine should be examined for evidence of spina bifida. Particular attention should be paid to the upper- and lowermost portions of the spine.

Skin

Note should be made of the tone of the skin, as well as the presence of any congenital birthmarks. Particular note should be made of the face, scalp, posterior neck, and sacral spine.

Extremities

All extremities should be examined for symmetry and shape. Note should be made of muscle tone and symmetry of movement and normal posture. Hips should be examined for evidence of hip dysplasia via the Barlow and Ortolani tests. The Barlow test is performed with the hips flexed to 90° and adducted. Downward pressure is applied to the knees. In infants with unstable hips, an audible and/or palpable click is noted. The Ortolani test is performed with the hips flexed to 90°. The hips are then gently adducted and then abducted. Again, note is made of an audible and/ or palpable click.

Neurologic

In addition to general responsiveness, tone, and activity, the neurologic examination may include evaluation of newborn reflexes. The Babinski reflex (or Babinski's sign) is generally present with dorsiflexion of toes in response to stimulation of the sole. Other reflexes that may be noted include grasping, rooting, and Moro. Moro reflex is characterized by abduction (spreading) and then adduction (pulling in) of the arms in response to a startling stimulus. Grasp reflex causes flexion of fingers in response to palmar stimulation. Rooting is noted when the infant turns its head in response to stroking of the cheek (turns toward).

Laboratory and Diagnostic Studies

All states mandate routine neonatal screening for a variety (between 26 and 40 unique diseases depending on state regulations) of abnormalities, including phenylalanine and thyroid-related disease and hemoglobinopathies. When appropriate, newborns will also be screened for syphilis and hyperbilirubinemia. Additional laboratory studies may be indicated based on the prenatal and maternal history. Most newborns will also undergo a newborn hearing screen.

All newborns should be evaluated for hearing prior to 1 month of age. This will often happen in the hospital prior to discharge. Screening examination is via one of two methods: (1) automated auditory brainstem response or (2) otoacoustic emissions test.

Newborns are almost universally screened for congenital heart disease at 24 h via pulse oximetry. A positive screening test may warrant echocardiography follow-up.

Vaccination

Most children will have received the first hepatitis B vaccine prior to discharge from the newborn nursery. Providers should confirm that this occurred.

Chapter 32
Routine Hospital Postpartum Management

Contents

Background... 225
Postpartum Day 1... 226
   History.. 226
   Physical Examination.. 226
   Laboratory Studies... 227
Management... 227
Postpartum Day 2... 228
   History.. 228
   Physical Examination.. 228
Laboratory Studies... 229
Management... 229

> **Key Points**
> 1. Postpartum management serves to identify early complications, if any, of the postpartum period.
> 2. Postpartum management includes educational as well as medical components.
> 3. Preconception management may begin in the immediate postpartum period.

Background

Immediate postpartum management falls largely within the domain of labor management and was discussed in detail in Chap. 19. The postpartum management of patients serves to identify early complications of the postpartum period as well as providing the basis for ongoing management of both the mother and new infant.

© Springer Nature Switzerland AG 2020
P. Lyons, N. McLaughlin, *Obstetrics in Family Medicine*, Current Clinical Practice,
https://doi.org/10.1007/978-3-030-39888-0_32

Postpartum Day 1

History

Evaluation on postpartum day 1 should begin with a brief review of the prenatal and labor and delivery course. Particular attention should be paid to those issues that may impact immediate postpartum care. Maternal laboratory values from the prenatal period should be reviewed. Particular note should be made of Rh status, maternal infection (urinary tract infections, sexually transmitted disease, and rubella and varicella immune status). Medical complications of pregnancy, such as hypertension, diabetes, and infection, should be noted.

Complications of delivery including prolonged labor and delivery method and immediate postpartum complications such as hemorrhage, uterine atony, or maternal fever should be reviewed. The management of these conditions and current status of each should be noted.

A variety of medical conditions such as an abnormal Pap smear may be uncovered in the prenatal course of management. These conditions will usually be deferred until after pregnancy. When present, these medical conditions should be noted. In addition, the management of a variety of medical conditions may have been modified during the course of pregnancy. Examples of this might include a change in hypertension medication or the discontinuation of antiseizure medications. When such changes have been made, the postpartum history should include prepregnancy treatment management as well as the management regimen implemented during pregnancy.

The history of postpartum day 1 focuses on a few key elements. Bowel and bladder function should be reviewed. When present, pain location and severity should be noted. Patient activity, including ambulation, should be noted. Patients should be asked about bleeding, discharge per vagina, and subjective fever.

Physical Examination

The postpartum examination is comprehensive but focuses primarily on a few key elements. Vital signs should be reviewed for maternal tachycardia and blood pressure. In patients for whom fluid status is being monitored (e.g., those with pre-eclampsia or those who are postoperative), weight should be recorded daily. Cardiovascular examination should include a note of cardiac murmurs. Pulmonary examination should note the presence of rales, rhonchi, or wheezing.

The most important elements of the physical examination are the abdomen and the perineum. On abdominal examination, note should be made of the size and consistency of the uterus as well as any tenderness if present. In general, the uterus should feel firm and the fundal height should be at or below the umbilicus. For patients who underwent operative delivery, note should be made of the surgical wound status. In the perineum, the external genitalia should be examined for swelling and tenderness. For patients who had an episiotomy or laceration, the site of the repair should be noted.

On postpartum day 1, all patients will have both bleeding and discharge per vagina. Note should be made of the quantity and quality of the bleeding. Although the distinction between normal and abnormal bleeding postpartum is sometimes difficult to make, normal postpartum bleeding should, in general, be no more than heavy menstrual bleeding. Clots may be noted in the early postpartum course but should resolve relatively quickly. In addition to bleeding, all postpartum patients will have a normal discharge per vagina referred to as lochia. Lochia represents a mixture of decidual tissue and blood in varying contents that changes in a predictable manner over time. In the first 3–4 days postpartum, this lochia includes considerable red blood cells and therefore appears red (lochia rubra). On postpartum day 3 or 4, as bleeding diminishes, the lochia becomes more pale or straw colored. This is referred to as lochia serosa. As the quantity of discharge diminishes and the presence of leukocytes increases, the lochia becomes clear (lochia alba). Lochia alba is variable in quantity and may last up to 8 weeks postpartum.

Laboratory Studies

As noted, all prenatal laboratory values should be reviewed. In the postpartum period, key laboratory values include hemoglobin or hematocrit (to assess for anemia) and rapid plasma reagin test (if not performed near term). In patients with fever or other signs of possible infection, a complete blood count with differential may assist in evaluation. White blood cell count must be interpreted with caution as it is often elevated in the postpartum period even in the absence of infection. In addition, urine, blood, and wound cultures should be obtained when appropriate.

Management

In addition to those items just noted, management will consist of assessment of and education concerning newborn care. Newborns can be expected to perform five basic functions: sleeping, eating, crying, urinating, and defecating. In addition to noting the presence or absence of each, providers should educate new parents about normal expectations for each, signs or symptoms of concern in each area, and appropriate follow-up for such warning signs. Although it is beyond the scope of this chapter to discuss each of these in detail, a few basic facts should be noted. All infants can be expected to urinate within the first few hours of life and note should be made of the number of wet diapers. If questions arise concerning the adequacy of urine output, these diapers can be weighed to determine the quantity of urine produced. All infants can be expected to stool prior to discharge, although they may not have done so by the time of the first postpartum rounds. The initial stools consist of meconium, a grainy, green material with little or any odor. These will gradually transition to more typical stools as the infant increases oral intake of either breast milk or formula.

All infants cry and parents should be made aware of the fact that this is neither abnormal nor of significant concern as long as the infant can be consoled and assessment is made that possible infant needs (hunger, stool, comfort) are met. Infants can be expected to sleep up to 18 h each day. Parents should be made aware, however, that this likely represents short periods of sleeping interspersed with periods of being awake. That is to say, it will not feel to most parents as if their newborn is sleeping most of the time. Parents should be educated to sleep when their infants sleep in anticipation of being awake at times when they might not usually anticipate being awake.

In general, all mothers without a specific contraindication to breastfeeding should be encouraged to breastfeed their newborn. This may begin in the immediate postpartum period while the patient is still in the delivery room setting. Breastfeeding itself stimulates the production of breast milk and earlier initiation enhances the likelihood of success. In the first several days, the principle available breast product is colostrum rather than breast milk. Parents should be assured that this is sufficient for most infants' needs in the period prior to the onset of breast milk production. New mothers may benefit from the assistance of skilled teaching in the breastfeeding technique by nursing staff, specialized lactation consultants, physicians, or other family members with breastfeeding experience.

Postpartum Day 2

History

For most patients with uncomplicated vaginal deliveries, postpartum day 2 represents the day of discharge to home. In addition to the elements just reviewed, providers should inquire about arrangements for transportation home (many institutions will not allow discharge of an infant unless the parents have a car seat) and arrangements at home.

Physical Examination

The examination on postpartum day 2 is similar to that of the first day. Abnormal findings noted on day 1 should be reviewed and particular attention should be paid to those areas on day 2.

Laboratory Studies

In general, there are no additional laboratory studies necessary on postpartum day 2, unless prior abnormal values require follow-up.

Management

As noted, postpartum day 2 is often the day of discharge from the hospital. Management should focus on transition of care from the hospital setting to the home setting and any needs the patient may have in arranging for this transition.

Chapter 33
Complications of the Hospital Postpartum Period

Contents

Background... 231
Persistent Postpartum Hemorrhage... 231
Hypertension... 232
Thromboembolic Disease.. 232
Fever.. 232
Infection.. 233
   Endometritis.. 233
   Urinary Tract Infections... 234

> **Key Points**
> 1. Fever in the postpartum period may be a sign of significant infection.
> 2. Although maternal temperature elevation may be normal in the first 24 h, persistent, markedly elevated, or unexplained fevers must be evaluated.

Background

For most pregnancies, the postpartum period is uncomplicated, and the routine management is discussed in Chap. 30. Occasionally, however, the hospital postpartum period is complicated by a variety of developments. Among these complications, postpartum hemorrhage, fever, and infection are the most common. Postpartum hemorrhage is discussed in Chap. 28.

Persistent Postpartum Hemorrhage

Follow-up with all postpartum women should include assessment of bleeding. While all women will report light bleeding (that will in most cases taper during the

P. Lyons, N. McLaughlin, *Obstetrics in Family Medicine*, Current Clinical Practice,
https://doi.org/10.1007/978-3-030-39888-0_33

postpartum hospital course), approximately 2% of women will experience more significant bleeding. Management of acute postpartum hemorrhage is discussed in Chap. 29. Evaluation beyond the immediate post delivery period will reflect a similar set of diagnostic considerations and interventions. Further evaluation may include ultrasonography to assess for retained placental remnants. Persistent bleeding may warrant uterine curettage.

Hypertension

Patients with chronic hypertension should be closely monitored in the postpartum period with continuation of the antihypertensive regimen utilized during pregnancy. Discussion of the management of hypertension in pregnancy is discussed in detail in Chap. 15. Patients with hypertensive complications of pregnancy should also be closely monitored in the postpartum period. Although at risk for further complications up to 1 week following delivery, highest risk is during the first 48 h. Because of the persistent risk beyond the usual postpartum hospital stay, these patients should generally be scheduled for a follow-up office visit within 1 week of delivery.

Thromboembolic Disease

All patients are at increased risk for thromboembolic events (deep vein thrombosis and pulmonary embolus) in the postpartum period. Risk is higher postpartum than at any other time during pregnancy (approximately fivefold higher incidence postpartum than during pregnancy). This elevated risk may last up to 3 months following delivery. In the postpartum period, all women should be monitored for leg swelling (new onset; asymmetric), shortness of breath, and/or chest pain. In the postpartum period, the use of warfarin (when indicated) is generally considered safe.

Fever

A variety of conditions may contribute to an elevated maternal temperature, especially in the first 24 h following delivery. Many of these conditions do not require specific intervention and are not considered a true fever. Maternal fever in the postpartum period is defined as a temperature of 38 °C (100.4 °F) on two occasions at least 24 h apart.

True maternal fever is relatively common, occurring in up to 10% of all pregnancies. Risk factors for postpartum fever include preceding maternal infection, prolonged rupture of membranes, and operative delivery. Although most postpartum fever will have an identifiable and treatable etiology, postpartum infection contributes to approximately 5% of maternal deaths.

When infection is identified, most consist of mixed anaerobic and aerobic flora of the genitourinary and gastrointestinal tracts. Common organisms include staphylococcal and streptococcal species, *E. coli*, gonorrhea, *Gardnerella*, and mycoplasma. Because of the local trauma inherent in delivery, most women will demonstrate asymptomatic colonization in the immediate postpartum period. As noted, however, true infection occurs in only 10% or less of women. Sterility of the intrauterine cavity can generally be demonstrated within 1 month of delivery.

Infection

Postpartum infection is generally one of three conditions: endometritis, urinary tract infection (UTI), or wound infection of the laceration or episiotomy. Of these, endometritis is, by far, the most common. UTI and wound infection are considerably less common, although each must be considered in the postpartum patient with true fever.

Endometritis

Endometritis is defined as an infection of the endometrium. As noted earlier, colonization of the endometrium following delivery is almost universal, but infection following routine delivery is considerably less frequent (~10%). Risk factors that increase the likelihood of endometritis include operative delivery, prolonged rupture of membranes, prolonged labor, pre-existing maternal infection including preceding chorioamnionitis, manual manipulation, and internal monitoring during pregnancy (intrauterine pressure catheter or fetal scalp electrode).

The diagnosis is suspected in the presence of maternal fever with foul-smelling lochia. The uterus is generally soft and tender, and the patient may demonstrate cervical motion tenderness. Laboratory studies include a complete blood count with differential, blood cultures and a urinalysis (to exclude the possibility of an UTI). The white blood cell count may be elevated with endometritis, but patients without infection may also demonstrate elevations in white blood cell count up to 20,000. Bacteremia is present in up to 10% of patients with endometritis, making blood cultures useful if positive but less helpful if negative.

In general, endometritis may be caused by a variety of aerobic and anaerobic streptococcal species, Gram-negative coliforms, chlamydia, or mycoplasma. Treatment should include broad-spectrum intravenous antibiotics with activity against suspected organisms. One such regimen would include clindamycin (Gram-positive and anaerobic coverage) plus an aminoglycoside (Gram-negative coverage) plus ampicillin (if *Enterococcus* is suspected).

Urinary Tract Infections

The combination of considerable manipulation and bacterial seeding with the urinary stasis associated with late-stage pregnancy makes UTI in the postpartum period a relatively common occurrence. Approximately 3% of pregnancies will be complicated by postpartum UTI. Diagnosis is made via urinalysis and urine culture. Treatment is directed by culture results or presumptive treatment for common pathogens (*E. coli*, *Proteus mirabilis*, *S. saprophyticus*). UTI diagnosis and management are discussed in detail in Chap. 13.

Chapter 34
Postpartum Clinic Visit

Contents

Background.. 235
Postpartum Depression... 236
Infant Care and Feeding.. 236
Sexuality/Relationships... 237
Vaginal Bleeding... 237
Self-Care.. 237
Management of Complications.. 238
    Hypertensive Disorders... 238
    Gestational Diabetes.. 238

Key Points
1. Screening for postpartum depression is an essential part of the postpartum visit.
2. Breastfeeding can be a significant source of stress during the postpartum period, even for multiparous patients who have had success with breastfeeding with prior infants.
3. Birth control counseling and future pregnancy planning should be confirmed at the postpartum visit.

Background

For many new parents, the postpartum period, the first 12 weeks after delivery, is a time of learning. They are adjusting to life with their new or expanding family. Historically, postpartum care was thought of as a single visit at 4–6 weeks postpartum. Given the magnitude of change in a new mother's life, it is unlikely that a single visit can adequately address all concerns. Rather a series of visits, either in office or by phone, might better serve the purposes of both the mother and physician. A mnemonic involving any number of B's (from 5 to 8 or more) has been used to que the provider to address issues present in the postpartum period. Alternatively one can think of issues in a head to toe format; in either case, a systematic approach is best to ensure important topics are covered. This chapter is written to address the issues and concerns faced by mothers in the postpartum period and does not address the issues faced by adoptive parents, couples who have used a surrogate or other non-traditional couples, or individuals who find themselves in the role of parent. That isn't to say these issues don't deserve important discussion but rather that it is beyond the scope of this book.

Postpartum Depression

Postpartum depression is a serious illness and should be screened for in settings where there exists a mechanism for follow-up and treatment. Postpartum depression can go unrecognized if not looked for explicitly. 10–15% of postpartum women will experience this condition with up to 33% of those women experiencing symptoms during the prenatal period. The USPSTF recommends that women at high risk for postpartum depression (Table 34.1) be provided with counseling during the prenatal period. A validated tool such as the Edinburgh Postpartum Depression Scale or Patient Health Questionnaire 9 (PHQ-9) should be used for the screening. Once postpartum depression is diagnosed, treatment and close follow-up should be initiated.

Infant Care and Feeding

Breastfeeding can be a source of both great joy and frustration. There are many factors that can affect the success of breastfeeding; the two most influential items are maternal education and partner support. As mentioned in Chap. 3 of this book, early breastfeeding education of both the woman and her partner/support system can greatly increase both breastfeeding initiation and continuation rates. It is also important to provide early support, potentially by phone or in home visits, as early frustra-

Table 34.1 Risk factors for postpartum depression	
	Personal or family history of depression
	Poor social support
	Family history of postpartum depression
	History of intimate partner violence/abuse
	Maternal or infant medical complications

tions are often causes of discontinuation of breastfeeding before the woman is even seen in the postpartum clinic setting. Also, it is important to understand the stress that can result from unsuccessful breastfeeding and to support the mother as best we can. While it is recognized that breastfeeding is superior to formula feeding in all but a few circumstances, maternal worth is not determined by the ability of a woman to breastfeed.

Sexuality/Relationships

A new addition to the family, whether it is the first infant or the fifth, forever alters the family landscape. In addition to prenatal counseling regarding sibling management and integration of the new baby into the family unit, it remains important to openly discuss family and intimate partner relationships, or the lack thereof, in the context of new parenting responsibilities. Relationships take work, and this certainly doesn't change in the postpartum setting. Resumption of sexual activity should also be addressed, and concerns related to this, including dyspareunia, can be addressed as needed. Continued discussions of birth control and future pregnancy planning should be undertaken as well and contraception adjusted to fit the needs of the patient.

Vaginal Bleeding

Normal lochia should progressively decrease in the days and weeks after discharge to a scant amount by 3–4 weeks. Persistent bleeding or an increase in bleeding should prompt an evaluation for retained placental parts. Fever could also signify other complications such as endometritis.

Self-Care

With the amount of effort that is required to raise an infant, it can be easy for the mother, or both parents frankly, to lose track of their own self-care, so it can be helpful for providers to bring it up as a topic of discussion. Sleep, of both the mother and the infant, is of paramount importance to both parties and can be a topic of great concern. It can be useful to help the mother to realize that there is no one right way to achieve good sleep for her and her infant, but rather a balance infant and maternal needs should be sought.

Management of Complications

Pregnancy and the postpartum period are times of physiologic flux and can be accompanied by a myriad of health conditions that require different follow-up routines. Below we will discuss some of the more common conditions and the key points of follow-up that should be addressed during the postpartum period.

Hypertensive Disorders

Whether pre-existing or related to pregnancy, hypertension necessitates close follow-up. A clinic visit with blood pressure measurement should be done within the first 7 days after discharge. Blood pressures of 160/110 or higher require inhospital management to prevent complications, including eclampsia. Lower measurements can be treated with antihypertensive medications suited to the individual patient. If hypertension persists beyond the postpartum period, then the patient should be transitioned to appropriate long-term antihypertensive agents with consideration of future pregnancy plans.

Gestational Diabetes

Gestational diabetes mellitus (GDM) increases the lifetime risk of the woman to develop type II diabetes mellitus by up to 20 times. It is therefore important to screen all women with GDM for impaired glucose tolerance in the postpartum period with a 75-gram 2 h glucose tolerance test. In addition a healthy diet and exercise should be encouraged during the postpartum period as they would be in any other patient.

Other issues can arise during pregnancy and the postpartum visit, including urinary incontinence and hemorrhoids, and should be addressed as appropriate.

Index

A

Abruptio placenta, 97–99
    placental abruption (*see* Placental
        abruption)
American College of Obstetrics and
        Gynecology (ACOG) guidelines, 27
Amniocentesis, 51
Assisted delivery
    cesarean section, 182
    curved blades, 180
    indications for forceps delivery, 181
    locking handles, 180
    low forceps, 181
    outlet forceps, 180
    use of forceps, 181
    vacuum-assist delivery, 181, 182

B

Babinski reflex, 223
β human chorionic gonadotropin (β-hCG), 83
Bleeding, 4
Brandt-Andrews maneuver, 210
Breastfeeding, 236

C

Carboprost, 211
Cesarean section, 182
Chorionic villus sampling (CVS), 52
Chromosomal abnormalities, 48

D

Diabetes mellitus (DM)
    classification, 136
    congenital abnormalities, 136

diagnosis, 136, 137
gestational diabetes
    management in labor, 141
    management in pregnancy, 140
    postpartum management, 141
    risk factors, 140
pregestational diabetes
    blood glucose monitoring, 139, 140
    diet, 138, 139
    educational interventions, 138
    first prenatal visit, 138
    insulin, 139
    oral hypoglycemics, 139
    preconception management, 137, 138
Dinoprostone, 170
Dizygotic (DZ) twins, 150
Down syndrome, 50

E

Early pregnancy bleeding
    differential diagnosis, 80
    ectopic pregnancy (*see* Ectopic
        pregnancy)
    etiology, 80
    evaluation and management, 80–82
    history, 81
    laboratory studies, 83
    physical examination, 81, 83
    spontaneous abortion (*see* Spontaneous
        abortion)
    ultrasound, 83
Ectopic pregnancy
    evaluation for, 85
    history, 84
    indications, 86

© Springer Nature Switzerland AG 2020
P. Lyons, N. McLaughlin, *Obstetrics in Family Medicine*, Current Clinical Practice,
https://doi.org/10.1007/978-3-030-39888-0

Ectopic pregnancy (*cont.*)
    intraperitoneal/extrauterine location, 84
    laboratory studies, 85
    medical management, 86
    patient stability, 85
    physical examination, 84, 85
    risk factors, 84
    surgical management, 86
    ultrasound, 85
Edinburgh Postpartum Depression Scale/
    Patient Health Questionnaire 9 item
    (PHQ-9), 236
Endometritis, 233, 234
Endometrium, 5
Epidural anesthesia, 175
Episiotomy, 213, 214
Estimated date of delivery (EDD), 66

F
Fertility
    hypothalamic function, 5, 6
    ovulation, 6, 7
    physiological conditions, 5
    pituitary function, 6
Fetal alcohol syndrome (FAS), 37
Fetal bradycardia, 199
Fetal heart rate monitoring
    acceleration, 199
    deceleration, 199
    early decelerations, 200
    fetal bradycardia, 199
    late decelerations, 200
    nonreassuring, 198
    routine fetal heart tracing, 198
    tachycardia, 199
    variable decelerations, 200
Fever, 232–233
Fibronectin, 67
First-degree lacerations, 215
Follicle-stimulating hormone (FSH), 5
Follicular development, 5
Follicular phase, 5
Food and Drug Administration (FDA), 38
Fourth-degree lacerations, 216

G
Gastrointestinal (GI) tract, 9
Genetic abnormality
    diagnosis, 49
    Down syndrome, 50
    history, 48, 49

neural tube defect
    amniocentesis, 51
    confirmation and diagnostic
      follow-up, 51
    CVS, 52
    physical examination, 49
    screening tests, 50
Genetic inheritance, 48
Gestational diabetes mellitus
    (GDM), 238
    management in labor, 141
    management in pregnancy, 140
    postpartum management, 141
    risk factors, 140
Gingival hypertrophy, 9
Gonadotropin-releasing hormone
    (GnRH), 6
Group B strep (GBS)
    diagnosis, 124, 125
    overview, 124
    screening, 125
    treatment, 125

H
Hepatitis B vaccine, 224
HIV
    antiretroviral use, 145, 146
    initial pregnancy evaluation, 144, 145
    intrapartum management, 146, 147
    postpartum management, 147
    preconception counseling, 144
Hospital postpartum period
    endometritis, 233, 234
    fever, 232–233
    hemorrhage, 231–232
    hypertension, 232
    thromboembolic disease, 232
    UTI, 234
Human chorionic gonadotropin (hCG)
    testing, 21
Hypertension
    chronic hypertension, 128, 131
    diagnosis, 128, 129
    history, 130
    laboratory studies, 130
    physical examination, 130
    pre-eclampsia, 128
      management of, 131–133
      postpartum management, 134
      prevention, 131
      seizure prevention, 133, 134
    risk factors, 129

I

Inactivated influenza vaccine (IIV), 42
Induction and augmentation
    contraindications, 169, 170
    indications for, 170
    mechanical options, 171
    oxytocin, 171
    prostaglandin formulations, 170
Infections
    antibiotics
        aminoglycosides, 118
        fluoroquinolones, 118
        safety and efficacy, 117
        sensitivity, 117
        sulfonamides, 117, 118
    fetal infection, 116, 117
    GBS
        diagnosis, 124, 125
        overview, 124
        screening, 125
        treatment, 125
    maternal, 115, 116
    symptoms, 115, 116
    UTIs
        bacterial seeding, 122
        diagnosis, 122
        history, 122, 123
        laboratory examination, 123
        physical examination, 123
        treatment, 123, 124
        urinary frequency, 122
    vaginitis/vaginosis
        complications, 119
        etiologic agents, 118
        gonorrhea/chlamydia, 121
        history, 119
        KOH, 120
        laboratory studies, 119
        microscopic examination, 120
        pH testing, 120
        physical examination, 119
        treatment, 120
        trichomoniasis, 121
        yeast vaginitis, 121
Intrauterine growth restriction (IUGR)
    complications, 57
    diagnosis, 60
    fetal growth assessment, 55
    management, risk reduction, 60–62
    risk factors, 54
        constitutional factors, 57
        fetal genetic, 55
        maternal factors, 56
        toxic exposures, 56, 57
        uterine environment, 55, 56

    screening for, 59
    SGA, 54, 55
    tracking fetal growth, 57–59

L

Laminaria, 171
Last menstrual period (LMP), 21, 24
Late-pregnancy bleeding
    differential diagnosis, 92
    evaluation, 93
    history, 94
    laboratory studies, 95
    physical examination, 95
    placenta previa (*see* Placenta previa)
    placental abruption (*see* Placental
        abruption)
    ultrasound, 94
Leopold's maneuvers, 76
Live Attenuated Influenza Vaccine (LAIV), 42
Local anesthesia, 175
Lochia, 227
Luteal cells, 5
Luteal phase, 5
Luteinizing hormone (LH), 5

M

Macrosomia, 159
Malpresentation
    breech presentation, 195
    compound presentation, 196
    incomplete breech, 195
    nonoccipital presentations, 194–195
    occipital position, 194
Maternal fever
    diagnostic studies, 205
    intraamniotic infection, 204
    management, 205
    physical examination, 204
    prenatal history, 204
Medications
    acetaminophen, 38
    acute medical conditions, 33
    acute obstetrical conditions, 34
    aspirin, 38
    chlorpheniramine, 39
    chronic medical conditions, 32, 33
    cough medications, 40
    decongestants, 39
    FAS, 37
    illicit drugs, 37
    NSAIDs, 39
    occupational exposures, 36
    OTC medications, 37, 38

Medications (*cont.*)
  principles, 32, 36
  proven human teratogens, 35, 36
  recommendations, 34
  tobacco, 36, 37
Menstruation, 4, 5
Methylergonovine, 211
Misoprostil, 211
Monozygotic (MZ) twins, 150
Multigestational pregnancy
  complications, 150
  diagnosis, 151
  DZ twins, 150
  history, 152
  labor and delivery, 153
  laboratory findings, 152
  MZ twins, 150
  physical examination, 152
  prenatal care, 152, 153

N
Narcotic analgesics, 34
Neural tube defect
  amniocentesis, 51
  confirmation and diagnostic follow-up, 51
  CVS, 52
Newborn evaluation
  abdomen, 222
  anus, 222
  cardiovascular, 221
  extremities, 223
  eyes, 221
  general observations, 221
  genital examination, 222
  head and neck, 221
  laboratory and diagnostic studies, 223–224
  neurologic, 223–224
  newborn history, 220
  physical examination, 220
  pulmonary/thoracic, 222
  skin, 223
  spine, 222
  vaccination, 224
  vital signs, 220
Nonsteroidal anti-inflammatory drugs
    (NSAIDs), 39
Normal labor
  Bishop scale cervical scoring, 164
  cervical dilation, 166
  effacement, 166
  history, 165
  laboratory studies, 167
  management, 167

  physical examination, 165
  prelabor, 164
  presentation, 166
  stages of, 165
  zero station, 166

O
Oligomenorrhea, 156
Oxytocin, 159, 160, 211

P
Pain management, labor
  nonpharmacological management, 174
  pharmacological management
    epidural–spinal anesthesia, 175–176
    local anesthesia, 175
    narcotic analgesics, 174, 175
Perineal lacerations, 214, 215
Placenta previa
  history, 96
  intravenous access sites, 97
  laboratory studies, 96
  management at term, 97
  overview, 95
  physical examination, 96
  preterm management, 97
  ultrasound, 96
Placental abruption
  history, 98
  laboratory studies, 99
  management
    mild abruption, 99
    moderate/severe abruption, 99, 100
    physical findings, 99
  maternal–fetal placental unit, 97
  physical examination, 98
  presentation for, 98
  ultrasound, 98
Postdates pregnancy
  amniotic fluid volume, 159
  assessment of fetal weight, 159
  biophysical profile scoring, 160
  contraction stress test, 159–160
  EDD, 156
  fetal kick count, 158
  fetal well-being, 157
  gestational age, 157
  gestational dating, 156
  management, 157, 158
  menstrual history, 156
  nonstress test, 159
  physical examination, 157

Postpartum clinic visit
  GDM, 238
  hypertensive disorders, 238
  infant care and feeding, 236–237
  postpartum depression, 236
  self care, 237
  sexuality/relationships, 237
  vaginal bleeding, 237
Postpartum depression, 236
Postpartum hemorrhage
  complications
    coagulopathy, 209
    lacerations, 209
    retained placenta, 209
    uterine atony, 208
    uterine fundus, 209
  definition, 208
  diagnosis, 209
  lacerations, 210
  management of, 210
  persistent bleeding, 211
Postpartum management
  day 1
    history, 226
    laboratory studies, 227
    management, 227, 228
    physical examination, 226–227
  day 2, 228, 229
Preconception counseling
  course of pregnancy, 11, 12
  education, 15, 16
  environmentally related factors, 13
  interventions, 16, 17
  patient-related factors, 12, 13
  pregnancy planning issue, 13, 14
  screening, 14–15
Pregnancy
  cardiovascular changes, 8
  gastrointestinal changes, 9
  hematological changes, 9
  physiological changes, 7
  renal/urinary changes, 8, 9
Premature rupture of membranes (PROM)
  history, 74, 75
  laboratory studies, 76
  management of, 77, 78
  overview, 73, 74
  physical examination, 75, 76
  risk factors, 74
Prenatal care
  diagnostic testing, 25, 26
  domains, 21, 22
  factors, 20

family history, 24
general medical history, 24
gestational age, 26, 27
interval studies, 29
laboratory testing, 25–27
LMP, 24
menstrual history, 22, 23
physical examination, 25
prenatal visits
  first trimester, 28
  follow-up visits, 27, 28
  frequency of visits, 22, 23
  interval history, 28
  second trimester, 28
  third trimester, 29
prior obstetrical history, 23, 24
treatment, 27
Preterm labor
  definition, 64
  diagnosis, 66
  environmental factors, 65
  fetal lung maturation
    early delivery, 70
    FLM-TDx II, 71
    gestational age, 70, 71
    lecithin-to-sphingomyelin ratio, 71
    phosphatidylglycerol, 71
  history, 66
  laboratory values, 67
  management, 67–70
  patient-related factors, 65, 66
  physical examination, 67
  risk factors, 64
Preterm premature rupture of membranes
  (PPROM), 65
Prolonged labor
  complications of, 184
  history, 185, 186
  laboratory/diagnostic studies, 185, 187,
    188
  latent-phase labor, 184
  management, 185, 186
  physical examination, 185–187

R
Recurrent pregnancy loss
  diagnosis, 103
  diagnostic studies, 104, 105
  history, 103, 104
  management, 103
  physical examination, 104
  risk factors, 102

Rh isoimmunization
    ABO blood type, 108
    diagnostic studies, 109
    evaluation and management, 110, 111
    for fetus, 108
    for infants, 109
    history, 109
    maternal–fetal transfusion, 110
    physical examination, 109
    potential sources, 110, 112
    Rh-negative patients, 108
    Rh-positive blood, 108
    Rh-sensitized mothers
        amniotic fluid assessment, 112
        critical threshold, 110
        postpartum monitoring, 110
        skilled maternal–fetal medicine
            provider, 110
        ultrasonography, 112
        umbilical sampling, 112

S
Second-degree lacerations, 215
Sexually transmitted disease (STD), 103
Shoulder dystocia
    clinical diagnosis, 190, 191
    complications of, 190
    management of, 191, 192
    maternal symphysis pubis, 189
    risk factors, 190
Small for gestational age (SGA), 54, 55
Spontaneous abortion
    complete abortion, 87, 89
    history, 87
    incomplete abortion, 87–89
    laboratory studies, 88
    overview, 86
    physical examination, 88
    risk factors, 87
    threatened abortion, 87, 88
    ultrasound, 88

T
Tachycardia, 199
Teratogenicity, 35
Tetanus, diphtheria and pertussis
        (Tdap), 43
Third-degree lacerations, 216
Thromboembolic disease, 232
Tocolysis, 69
Tranexamic acid, 211

U
Urinary tract infections (UTIs), 234
    bacterial seeding, 122
    diagnosis, 122
    history, 122, 123
    laboratory examination, 123
    physical examination, 123
    treatment, 123, 124
    urinary frequency, 122
Uterine massage, 211

V
Vaccination in pregnancy
    guidelines, 44
    hepatitis A, 43
    infections, 42
    influenza, 42
    meningococcal B strain, 43
    recommendations, 42
    Tdap, 43
    yellow fever, 43
    zoster, 44

Z
Zero station, 166

Printed in the United States
By Bookmasters